Here's what readers had to say about the G.I. Diet:

"The G.I. Diet has done what I considered to be the impossible. When I first started it, I weighed well over 200 pounds. Twenty weeks later, I reached 168 pounds! That's over 30 pounds! Needless to say, my pants have all gone to charity and I've had to buy new ones two sizes smaller. I have a healthy BMI, healthy waistline, feel great and I'm maintaining the weight. I'll continue this program for the rest of my life." — James

"I can't believe that after two pregnancies and at the age of 32, I weigh what I did in high school! It's thanks to the G.I. Diet! I've tried other diets but this is the one that has changed the way I eat and exercise for life . . . I have never felt better, more active and more energetic. What a joy to be able to go on long hikes, canoe trips and bike rides with my husband and feel terrific doing it!" — Janine

"Wow! It has been seven months since I started the diet and I have lost 72 pounds! What a great feeling. I can go shopping again and not be embarrassed about the size I buy . . . It is such a new way to live and I love it. So many people have commented on the way I look. My husband is so happy about the results, he has started on the program." — Catherine

"I have been overweight all my life. . . . I peaked at 302 pounds and came to the conclusion that I was a food addict and that trying to lose weight was hopeless, having tried and failed with every other plan out there—or so I thought! Thank God, a very dear friend of mine found *The G.I. Diet*. Seven weeks later I weigh 273 pounds and have never felt so good . . . I KNOW I am going to get down to a healthy body weight for the first time in my life." — Sarah

"I'm absolutely amazed at the progress I have made in reducing my cholesterol level. Before starting the G.I. Diet, my cholesterol was 6.9 and slowly increasing . . . Ten short weeks later, by following the G.I. Diet to the letter, my cholesterol level is now 4.62. Even my doctor is astounded, because I have NEVER been below 5 on a cholesterol test. I'm a believer . . . the G.I. Diet gets results in short order." — Robert

"To date, I have lost 25 pounds and my wife has lost 15 pounds. We are almost back to where we were on our wedding day forty-two years ago. We have no doubt that we will be able to keep it off for good." — Ray

"I have tried several diet plans, but none worked for any length of time—all the weight I lost came back three-fold . . . Then I went out and purchased *The G.I. Diet* and began to read it . . . Since then I have lost a total of 63 pounds and have dropped from a size 28 (which was a very tight 28) to a size 18! More important than the weight loss is the fact that my last blood work done by my doctor was unbelievable—my cholesterol levels have dropped drastically, and I am now in the normal levels! . . . This G.I. Diet is the best!" — Pamela

"I was 240 pounds eight weeks ago. I'm now down to 210 pounds and amazingly I have dropped two dress sizes. The weird thing is, apart from relinquishing the obligatory spud at every meal, I still feel like I've yet to start the diet! I feel absolutely wonderful. . . . And my husband can't keep his hands off me! My doctor is stunned by my progress and is going to start recommending *The G.I. Diet* to his other obese patients." — Maeve

"I have had much success with the G.I. Diet. Last week I bought some trousers with a 34-inch-waist—the first of that size that I have been able to wear since I was 27 years old, thirty-three years ago . . . The weight loss rate has been phenomenal. This is the first simple intelligent diet that I have ever seen." — Mike

"Both my husband, who has lost almost 50 pounds, and I, who lost almost 15 pounds, are totally in awe of this new lifestyle. We just love how sensible and easy it is to follow." — Julia

"I put on 40 pounds after my pregnancy and was plagued with severe fatigue and muscle pain. . . . Within a short time on the G.I. Diet, my energy level increased and I started to feel better. Since then I've lost about 26 pounds (with 20 more to lose by the end of this year). My waist alone has decreased from about 41 inches to 33 1/2 inches. . . . Most importantly, I feel great!" — Anita

"I have dropped 54 pounds over the last twelve months and am on my way to a BMI of 22. I will be there by the time the hot weather hits in June. I don't feel like I'm on a diet, and have even taken some 'holidays.' I have never felt better! It's a whole new life!" — Linda

"I am 5'9" and started the diet at 219 pounds. Well, I am happy to say that as of 5:30 this morning, I hit the scales at 168 pounds! The G.I. Diet is not so much a diet as it is a change in lifestyle." — Kevin

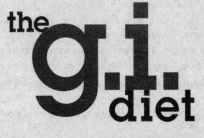

the g.i. diet

THE EASY, HEALTHY WAY
TO PERMANENT WEIGHT LOSS

RICK GALLOP

Past President of the Heart & Stroke Foundation of Ontario

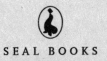

SEAL BOOKS

Seal Books and colophon are trademarks of Random House of
Canada Limited.

THE G.I. DIET
Seal Books/published by arrangement with Random House Canada
Random House Canada edition published 2002
Seal Books edition published December 2003

ISBN 0-7704-2954-8

Cover design: Carol Moskot
Interior design: Jean Lightfoot Peters
Printed and bound in the USA

Seal Books are published by Random House of Canada Limited.
"Seal Books" and the portrayal of a seal are the property of
Random House of Canada Limited.

Visit Random House of Canada Limited's website:
www.randomhouse.ca

OPM   10   9   8   7   6   5   4   3   2   1

Contents

Foreword

It's hard to ignore, especially as a cardiologist, the fact that obesity has ballooned into a crisis of epidemic proportions in North America. It affects one in three adults and one in four children and teenagers. In my own practice, I see a disproportionate number of patients who are overweight or obese, as obesity is a recognized risk factor for conditions that are the foundations for heart attack and stroke. Contrary to popular belief, abdominal fat is not merely a passive repository of excess weight; it is actively associated with hormones that endanger health. A waist circumference of greater than 36 inches (90 centimetres) is associated with a high-risk profile for coronary heart disease.

Millions of people are on diets, spending billions of dollars on self-help, quick-fix books, weight loss programs, diet drinks and foods. The continued growth of the weight loss industry is assured since so many of these plans and practices fail in the face of unachievable expectations. Indeed, many dieters rebound to weights exceeding their original. Obesity is a chronic condition, and effective weight management requires a long-term behavioural strategy. The promises of easy weight loss diets are false and will not result in long-term success. The marked early weight loss seen in high protein diets, for example, is due to water loss, not fat loss, because high protein intake is dehydrating. The typical dieter is doomed to repeat failure because he or she chases the fantasy of a dream weight and a fast solution rather than learns from experience and finally confronts the reality of achievable, permanent weight loss. The laws of thermodynamics are irrefutable, even for dieters: to lose one pound of fat you must achieve a deficit of 3,600 calories.

An often forgotten element of weight loss and long-term weight control is exercise. Aerobic exercise not only burns calories (albeit modestly) but also improves cardio-vascular conditioning and reduces cardiac risk. Finally, exercise seems to have a magical effect on the dieter: it reduces appetite, and the feeling of body tone seems to act as a food traffic signal at mealtime.

Why read *The G.I. Diet*, another book on a long shelf of "New You" promises? If you want weight loss fiction, this book isn't for you. *The G.I. Diet* is an innovative, realistic, uncomplicated, long-term approach to successful weight management. To create this diet, Rick Gallop has drawn on his long experience with the Heart and Stroke Foundation of Ontario and its research and public educa-tion programs. He discusses the principles of nutrition and illustrates these with anecdotes and humour, which bring them alive and make them easy to digest.

Building on this practical knowledge, Rick then tackles the problem of weight loss as a long-term issue, leading you through the supportive elements of behavioural change, including the development of achievable specific goals: How much should I lose per week? Exactly how will I do it? If I fail one day, how do I respond? How do I cope with breakfast meetings, luncheon meetings, muffins in midday meetings, and then fast-food dinners or more formal dinners out? You only live once and food is one of life's great pleasures. Counting calories is not a preferred option.

The G.I. Diet presents the reader with a simple guide to food choices, both at home and away, with easy-to-remember images, practical tips, tasty recipes and strategies for feedback and self-monitoring. The critical importance of exercise is also addressed. Finally, Rick Gallop has included an assortment of self-help weight loss tools—additions that the reader is certain to find useful.

With a heavy travel schedule, lunchtime meetings and dinners out, I must be continually vigilant about my weight. The principles and ideas described by Rick Gallop in this book have certainly been beneficial to me. *The G.I. Diet* charts a course that if followed will deliver its promise of permanent weight loss.

Michael J. Sole, MD, FRCP(C); FACC
Former Chief of Cardiology, The Toronto Hospital
Professor of Medicine and Physiology
Founder of The Centre for Cardiovascular Research,
University of Toronto

Introduction

While I was president of the Heart and Stroke Foundation of Ontario for fifteen years, my job was to raise funds for research into heart disease and stroke and to promote healthy lifestyle choices among Canadians to reduce their risk for those diseases. The Foundation has developed the most comprehensive set of heart disease, stroke and healthy lifestyle resources in Canada. We now know that smoking, high blood pressure, high blood cholesterol, a sedentary lifestyle and being overweight are all major risk factors for heart attacks and strokes. So a few years ago, when I was twenty pounds overweight, I knew I had to reduce. And with all the information and resources I had, I thought I knew how: I went out and bought a Nordic ski machine and a stationary bike, and I started working out every day. But however hard I exercised, I found I could only stabilize, not lose, the weight. For the first time in my life, I realized I had to go on a diet.

Conventional nutritional wisdom at the time recommended a low-fat, high-carbohydrate diet. All I had to do was stop eating fatty foods like cheese and ice cream, and start eating more low-fat carbohydrates like pasta, rice and vegetables—right? Wrong. Though I stuck diligently to the diet, eating pasta and tomato sauce instead of steak and Caesar salad, I wasn't losing any weight at all. In frustration, I turned to the filing cabinets at the Heart and Stroke Foundation of Ontario. The Foundation receives literally hundreds of diet books, products and recipes every year, all hoping for support or endorsement. Looking through the files, I quickly ruled out food-specific diets, such as the grapefruit or banana diet, because they have no scientific basis, are risky to your health, and are impossible to sustain over the long term.

I also decided to avoid high-protein diets since various studies had found them to be a real health hazard. High-protein diets, which drastically limit the amount of carbohydrates you consume, put the body in a state of ketosis. As the body is starved of carbohydrates, your principal source of energy, it starts breaking down protein, including the body's own lean muscle, for energy, which releases a lot of water weight. This creates toxic by-products called ketones, which are removed from the body through the kidneys and can cause an array of problems, from mild nuisances like bad breath to toxic side effects such as kidney damage, diarrhea, dizziness and kidney stones. And because so much protein blocks calcium absorption, people who follow high-protein diets develop bone weakness too. To complete this tale of woe, when you go off the diet, the water weight loss is quickly replaced, and unless you are into a heavy exercise regimen, the weight you gain back will all be fat; the muscle loss will not be recovered.

So, diets based on a single food, and high-protein diets were out. I was still left with a whole host of diets to try, and I selected one that appeared to be based on sound nutritional principles. After several unsuccessful months with that one, I embarked on another, and then a few months later, another. In the end I tried I don't know *how* many of them. I counted calories. I studied labels—a real challenge with Canadian labelling regulations (or lack thereof). I starved. I hallucinated about food. Sometimes I did lose a few pounds, but then I'd hit the inevitable plateau, unable to go any further. And since I was constantly hungry, I'd soon start eating what I wanted and gain back the few pounds I'd managed to lose.

It seemed like I was destined to spend the rest of my life overweight. It was the most discouraging thing I have ever experienced. I couldn't understand why losing weight was so difficult, and I felt there had to be a way to slim down and maintain a healthy weight without having to feel hungry every moment of the day, jeopardizing one's health or requiring a Ph.D. in math to calculate various formulas and ratios. I was determined to find a diet that would work, not only for myself but also for others in the same boat—gaining weight and increasing their risk for heart disease and stroke, not to mention diabetes.

My quest eventually led me to one of the nutritional researchers supported by the Heart and Stroke Foundation of Ontario. He introduced me to the G.I., or Glycemic Index, through a book called *The Zone* by Dr. Barry Sears. *The Zone* diet is based on the principles of the G.I., which measures the speed at which your body breaks down carbohydrates and converts them to glucose, the vehicle your body uses for energy. The faster the food breaks down, the higher the rating on the index. When trying to lose weight it is critical to avoid foods that have a high G.I. and to eat low-G.I. foods instead. The glycemic index was invented by Dr. David Jenkins, a professor of nutrition at the University of Toronto. Since he was living in my hometown, I decided to pay him a visit.

A lean Englishman who clearly practises what he preaches, Dr. Jenkins explained that early in his research career he became interested in diabetes, a disease that hampers the body's ability to process carbohydrates and sugar (glucose). Sugar therefore stays in the bloodstream instead of going into the cells, resulting in hyperglycemia and potentially coma. At the time Dr. Jenkins was beginning his research, carbohydrates were severely restricted in a diabetic's diet as they quickly boost the sugar level in the bloodstream. But because the primary role of carbohydrates is to provide the body with energy, diabetics were having to make up the lack of calories through a high-fat diet, which does not boost sugar levels. As a result, many diabetics were increasingly at risk of dying from heart disease, since fat is a critical factor in the development of that disease. Doctors were in a real quandary: although they were saving diabetics from starvation, they were accelerating their risk of heart disease.

Dr. Jenkins wondered if all carbohydrates are the same. Are some digested more quickly and as a result raise blood sugar levels faster than others? And are others "slow-release," resulting in only a marginal increase in blood sugar? The answer, Jenkins discovered, is yes. He published an index—the glycemic index—in 1980, showing the various rates at which carbohydrates break down and release glucose into the bloodstream.

I decided to try *The Zone*. To my amazement and delight I lost the twenty pounds that had been plaguing me for so long. I invited some of my friends and associates to try it as well. By the end of twelve months, however, 95 percent had dropped out. They cited two principal reasons for their inability to stick to the diet: 1) it was too complex for everyday life, requiring them to count grams and calculate formulas and ratios; and 2) they were always feeling hungry, which is the death knell for any diet.

The 5 percent who managed to hang in were so happy with their success that I received numerous e-mails from them describing how important their weight control was in their lives. Here are a few of their comments:

Overall, I have lost twenty-two pounds. And I feel more energized . . . I don't even notice that I'm eating differently. I certainly don't feel like I'm on a diet; I just feel like I eat in a new way.

Well, with Thanksgiving, two large family dinners, weekend guests, lunches with friends, being on the road and my love of wine and food, I have managed to lose fifteen pounds. I can honestly say my energy is better—I'm not falling asleep in front of the TV any more.

This weekend, my son returns home from univer-
sity to attend his commencement ceremonies at
his high school. After fourteen years, I will be
wearing the same skirt I wore when I dropped
him off for his first day of school in Grade 1.

Dismayed by the 95 percent dropout rate but bolstered by the successful 5 percent, I set out to address the two key impediments to success: complexity and hunger. The result is this book. The G.I. Diet is simple to follow and will not leave you feeling hungry. The plan comprises a unique combination of foods that have two essential characteristics: they make you feel full for a longer time, so you are naturally inclined to eat less, and they are low-calorie. If you, like me, have been reading other recent diet books, you will have noticed that the word *calorie* is never used. But lowering caloric intake is the only route to weight loss, and all those diets are, in fact, low-calorie; it's just that the word has been omitted. With the G.I. Diet, you won't need to count calories, or weigh or measure your food. I've done all the math for you to create the easiest eating plan possible, one that reflects the demands of the busy world we live in. While most diet books take three hundred pages or more to make their point, *The G.I. Diet* is simple and concise, with very little scientific jargon. Its most important feature is that *it works.* You'll find it so simple to follow, so effective, you'll never have to pick up a diet book again.

CHAPTER ONE

The Problem

While I was waging my personal battle of the bulge, I couldn't help but be struck by the number of people who were engaged in the same struggle. The statistics are truly astonishing: 50 percent of Canadian adults today are overweight. That's more than double what it was only ten years ago. What's happened to us? Why have we gained so much weight in the last decade?

The simple explanation is that people are eating too many calories. Unless one denies the basic laws of thermodynamics, the equation never changes: consume more calories than you expend and the surplus is stored in the body as fat. That's the inescapable fact. But that doesn't explain why people today are eating more calories than they used to. To answer that question we must first understand the three key components of any diet—carbohydrates, fats and proteins—and how they work in our digestive system. Since fats are probably the least understood part, let's start with them.

Fats

Fat is definitely a bad word these days, and it engenders an enormous amount of confusion and contradiction. But are you aware that fats are absolutely essential to your diet? They contain various key elements that are crucial to the digestive process.

The next fact might also surprise you: fat does not necessarily make you fat. The quantity you consume does. And that's something that's often difficult to control, because your body *loves* fat. Non-fat foods require lots of processing to be transformed into those fat cells around your waist and hips; fatty foods just slide right in. Processing takes energy, and your body hates wasting energy. It needs to expend about 20 to 25 percent of the energy it gets from a non-fat food just to process it. So your body definitely prefers fat, and as we all know from personal experience, it will do everything it can to persuade us to eat more of it. That's why fatty foods like juicy steaks, chocolate, and decadent ice creams taste so good to us. But because fat contains twice as many calories per gram as carbohydrates and proteins, we really have to be careful about the amount of fat we eat.

In addition to limiting *how much* fat we consume, we must also pay attention to the *type* of fat. While the type of fat has no effect on our weight, it is critical to our health—especially heart health.

There are four types of fat: the best, the better, the bad and the really ugly. The "bad" fats are called saturated fats, and they are easily recognizable because they almost always come from animal sources and they solidify at room temperature. Butter, cheese and meat are all high in saturated fats. There are a couple of others you should be aware of too: coconut oil and palm oil are two vegetable oils that are saturated, and because they are cheap, they are used in many snack foods, especially cookies. Saturated fats are a principal cause of heart disease because they boost cholesterol, which in turn thickens arteries and causes heart attack and stroke.

Fifteen years ago a wealthy American industrialist had a heart attack. Like many successful businessmen he hated surprises, and he wanted to know what had caused the unexpected turn in his health. When he discovered that many leading food products contain tropical oils such as palm and coconut, he took out a full-page ad in *The Wall Street Journal* declaring: "THESE 9 PRODUCTS ARE KILLING AMERICANS." Within forty-eight hours, eight of the nine products were reformulated without the tropical oils. Check your labels.

The "really ugly" fats are potentially the most dangerous. They are vegetable oils that have been heat-treated to make them thicken. These hydrogenated oils take on the worst characteristics of saturated fats, so don't use them, and avoid snack foods, baked goods and cereals that contain them. Check the label for "hydrogenated oils" or "partially hydrogenated oils."

The "better" fats are called polyunsaturated, and they are cholesterol free. Most vegetable oils, such as corn and sunflower, fall into this category. What you should really be using, however, are monounsaturated fats, the "best," which are found in olives, peanuts, almonds, and olive and canola oils. Monounsaturated fats have a beneficial effect on cholesterol and are good for your heart. (See chapter 9 for more information on cholesterol and heart disease.) Though fancy olive oils are expensive, you can get the same health benefits from reasonably priced house brands at your supermarket. Olive oil is used extensively in the famed Mediterranean diet, which is also rich in fruits and vegetables. Because of their diet, southern Europeans have some of the lowest rates of heart disease in the world, and obesity is not a problem in those countries. So look for monounsaturated fats and oils on food labels. Most manufacturers who use them will say so, because they know it's a key selling point for informed consumers.

Another highly beneficial oil, which is in a category of its own, contains a wonderful ingredient called omega-3. This oil is found in deep-sea fish such as salmon and in flax and canola seed. It's extremely good for your heart health (see page 130).

So we know that it's important to avoid the bad and the really ugly fats and to incorporate the best fats in our diets to make our hearts healthy. Many of us have tried to lower our fat intake by using leaner cuts of meat and drinking lower-fat milk. But even with these modifications our fat consumption hasn't decreased. Why? Because many of our favourite foods—like crackers, muffins, cereals and fast foods—contain hidden fats. Detecting them often seems to require an advanced degree in nutrition, since labelling of nutritional components has been voluntary in Canada (unlike the U.S.). A good rule of thumb is to avoid any food whose package does not list its nutritional components; this usually means that the manufacturer has something to hide.

COOKING OILS/FATS

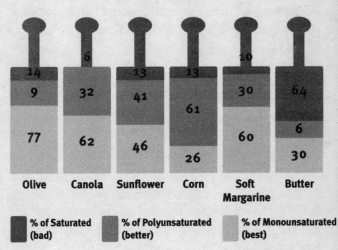

| | % of Saturated (bad) | % of Polyunsaturated (better) | % of Monounsaturated (best) |

So we're not eating less fat, but contrary to popular belief, neither are we eating more. Fat consumption in this country has remained virtually constant over the past ten years, while obesity numbers have doubled. Obviously, fat isn't the culprit. What has increased is our consumption of *grain*. Grain is a carbohydrate, so let's look at how carbohydrates work.

TO SUM UP:
1. Eat less fat overall and look for low-fat alternatives to your current diet.
2. Eat monounsaturated and polyunsaturated fats only.

Carbohydrates

Carbohydrates are the primary source of energy for your body. They are found in grains, vegetables, fruits, legumes and dairy products. Your body takes in carbohydrates from these foods and converts them into glucose. The glucose dissolves in your bloodstream and is diverted to those parts of your body that use energy, like your muscles and your brain. (It may surprise you to know that when you are resting your brain uses about two-thirds of the glucose in your system!)

Carbohydrates, obviously, are essential for your body to function. They are rich in fibre, vitamins and minerals, including antioxidants, which we now believe play a critical role in protecting against disease, especially heart disease and cancer. For years we've been advised by doctors, nutritionists and government to eat a low-fat, high-carbohydrate diet, and grains form the base of Canada's Food Guide. The trouble with this is that it has encouraged us all to rely too much on them. Just look at the amount of space dedicated to grain-based products in our supermarkets today: huge cracker, cookie and snack food sections; whole aisles of cereals; numerous shelves of pastas and noodles; and baskets and baskets of bagels, rolls, muffins and loaves of bread. I can remember when bagels were exclusive to the Jewish community; now most food stores carry half a dozen different varieties, and chains of bagel stores are spread across the country. Muffins were never as abundant as they are today. (Not so very long ago, a colleague of mine was coming in to work bleary-eyed every day. When I asked her what was happening, she explained that she was staying up each night baking different flavoured muffins for a new retail idea of her husband, Michael Bregman. He went on to found the mmmuffins chain—and the rest, as they say, is history.)

Another modern food sensation has been pasta, once viewed as an ethnic specialty in North America. That's hard to believe today, with pasta a staple on most restaurant menus and every family's shopping list. Eighty percent of Canadian homes now serve pasta at least once a week. And our snack-food options have multiplied: crackers, tortilla

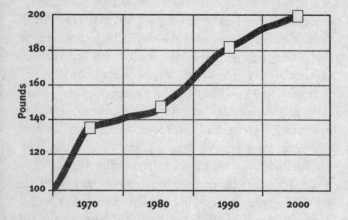

GRAIN CONSUMPTION (pounds per capita)

Source: U.S. Department of Agriculture

chips, corn chips, pretzels and countless varieties of cookies, to name just a few.

In 1970 the average North American ate about 135 pounds of grain. By 2000 that figure had risen to about 200 pounds. That's a 50-percent increase! Why should we be concerned about this? Aren't wheat, corn and rice low-fat? How could grain be making us fat?

The answer lies in the *type* of grain we're eating today, most of which is in the form of white flour. White flour starts off as whole wheat. At the mill the whole wheat is steamed and scarified by tiny razor-sharp blades to remove the bran, or outer shell, and the endosperm, the next layer. Then the wheat germ and oil are removed because they turn rancid too quickly to be considered commercially viable. What's left after all that processing is unbleached flour, which is then whitened and used to make almost all the breads, bagels, muffins, cookies, crackers, cereals and pastas we consume. Even many "brown" breads are simply artificially coloured white bread.

It's not just grain that's highly processed nowadays. A hundred years ago most of the food people ate came straight from the farm to the dinner table. Lack of refrigeration and scant knowledge of food chemistry meant that most food remained in its original state. However, advances in science, along with the migration of many women out of the kitchen and into the workforce, led to a revolution in prepared foods. Everything became geared to speed and simplicity of preparation. Today's high-speed flour mills use steel rollers rather than the traditional grinding stones to produce an extraordinarily finely ground product, ideal for producing light and fluffy breads and pastries. We now have instant rice and potatoes, as well as entire meals that are ready to eat after just a few minutes in the microwave.

The trouble with all this is that the more a food is processed beyond its natural state, the less processing your body has to do to digest it. And the quicker you digest your food, the sooner you are hungry again, and the more you tend to eat. We all know the difference between eating a bowl of old-fashioned slow-cooking oatmeal and a bowl of sugary cold cereal. The oatmeal stays with you—it "sticks to your ribs" as my mother used to say—whereas you are looking for your next meal an hour after eating the bowl of sugary cereal. That's why our ancestors did not have the obesity problem we have today; their foods were basically unprocessed and natural. All the great food companies, like Kraft, General Foods, Kellogg's, McCain, Nabisco and Del Monte, only started processing and packaging natural foods in the past century or so.

Our fundamental problem, then, is that we are eating foods that are too easily digested by our bodies. Clearly, we can't wind back the clock to simpler times, but we need somehow to slow down the digestive process so we feel hungry less often. How can we do that? Well, we have to eat foods that are "slow-release," that break down at a slow and steady rate in our digestive system, leaving us feeling fuller for longer.

How do we identify those "slow-release" foods? There are two clues. The first is the amount of fibre in the food. Fibre, in simple terms, provides low-calorie filler. It does double duty, in fact: it literally fills up your stomach, so you feel satiated; and your body takes much longer to break it down, so it stays with you longer and slows down the digestive process. There are two forms of fibre: soluble and insoluble. Soluble fibre is found in foods like oatmeal, beans, barley and citrus fruits, and has been shown to lower blood cholesterol levels. Insoluble fibre is important for normal bowel function and is typically found in whole wheat breads and cereals and most vegetables.

The second tool in identifying slow-release foods is the glycemic index, which I will now explain. It is the core of this diet and the key to successful weight management.

TO SUM UP:
Eat foods that have not been highly processed and that do not contain highly processed ingredients.

The Glycemic Index

The glycemic index measures the speed at which you digest food and convert it to glucose, your body's energy source. The faster the food breaks down, the higher the rating on the index. The index sets sugar (glucose) at 100 and scores all foods against that number. Here are some examples:

Baguette	95	Donut	76	Muffin (bran)	56	Oatmeal	42	Fettuccine	32
Instant Rice	87	Cheerios	75	Popcorn (low-fat)	55	Spaghetti	41	Beans	31
Baked Potatoes	84	Bagel	72	Orange	44	Apple	38	Grapefruit	25
Cornflakes	84	Raisins	64	All-Bran	43	Tomato	38	Fat- and sugar-free yogurt	14

The chart on the next page illustrates the impact of sugar on the level of glucose in your bloodstream compared with kidney beans, which have a low G.I. rating. As you can see, there is a dramatic difference between the two. Sugar is quickly converted into glucose, which dissolves in your bloodstream, spiking its glucose level. It also disappears quickly, leaving you wanting more. Have you ever eaten a large Chinese meal, with lots of noodles and rice, only to find yourself hungry again an hour or two later? That's because your body rapidly converted the rice and noodles, high-G.I. foods, to glucose, which then quickly disappeared from your bloodstream. Something most of us experience regularly is the feeling of lethargy that follows an hour or so after a fast-food lunch, which generally consists of high-G.I. foods. The surge of glucose followed by the rapid drain leaves us starved of energy. So what do we do? Around mid-afternoon we look for a quick sugar fix, or snack, to bring us out of the slump. A few cookies or a bag of chips cause another rush of glucose, which disappears a short time later—and so the vicious cycle continues. No wonder we're a nation of snackers!

When you eat a high-G.I. food and experience a rapid spike in blood sugar, your pancreas releases the hormone insulin. Insulin does two things extremely well. First, it reduces the level of glucose in your bloodstream by

G.I. IMPACT ON SUGAR LEVELS

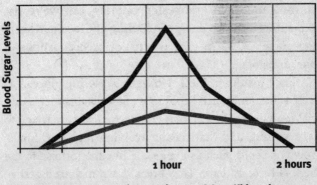

diverting it into various body tissues for immediate short-term use or by storing it as fat—which is why glucose disappears so quickly. Second, it inhibits the conversion of body fat back into glucose for the body to burn. This evolutionary feature is a throwback to the days when our ancestors were hunter-gatherers, habitually experiencing times of feast or famine. When food was in abundance, the body stored its surplus as fat to tide it over the inevitable days of famine. Insulin was the champion in this process, both helping to accumulate fat and then guarding its depletion.

Today, everything has changed except our stomachs. A digestive system that has taken millions of years to evolve is, in a comparative blink of an eye, expected to cope with a food revolution. We don't have to hunt and search for food any more; we have a guaranteed supply of highly processed foods with a multitude of tempting flavours and textures at the supermarket. Not only are we consuming more easily digested calories, but we're not expending as much energy in finding our food and keeping ourselves warm—the two major preoccupations of our ancestors.

Since insulin is the key trigger to storing glucose as well as the sentry that keeps those fat cells intact, it is crucial to maintain low insulin levels when you are trying to lose weight, and that means avoiding high-G.I. foods. Low-G.I. foods such as apples are like the tortoise to the high-G.I. foods' hare. They break down in your digestive system at a slow, steady rate. You don't get a quick sugar fix when you eat them, but, tortoiselike, they stay the course, so that you feel full longer. Therefore if you want to lose weight, you must stick to low-G.I. foods.

But the fact that a food has a low G.I. does not necessarily make it desirable. The other critical factor determining whether a food will allow us to lose weight is its calorie content. It's the combination of low-G.I foods with few calories, i.e., low in sugar and fat, that is the "magic bullet" of the G.I. Diet. Low-G.I., low-calorie foods make you feel more satiated than do foods with a high G.I. and calorie level. Later in this book I will provide you with a comprehensive chart identifying the foods that will make you fat and those that will allow you to lose weight. Don't expect all the low-G.I. foods to be tasteless and boring! There are many delicious and satisfying choices that will make you feel as though you aren't even on a diet.

I've already mentioned two of the principal factors that contribute to a food's G.I. rating: the degree of processing it undergoes before it is digested and how much fibre it contains. But there are two other important components that inhibit the rapid breakdown of food in our digestive system, and they are fat and protein. The influence of these two factors can lead to some surprising, and confusing, results. Peanut butter, for example, has a low G.I. because of its high fat and protein content. Similarly, whole milk has a lower G.I. than skim, and fruitcake has a lower G.I. than melba toast. Fat, like fibre, acts as a brake in the digestive process. When combined with other foods it becomes a barrier to digestive juices. It also signals the brain that you are satisfied and do not require more food. But we know that many fats are harmful to your heart, and they contain twice the number of calories per gram as carbohydrates and protein. Since protein also acts as a brake in the digestive process, let's look at it in more detail.

TO SUM UP:

1. Low-G.I. foods are slower to digest, so you feel satiated longer.
2. Keeping insulin levels low inhibits the formation of fat and assists in the conversion of fat back into energy.
3. The key to losing weight is to eat low-G.I., low-calorie foods.

Protein

As with fat, there's been a great deal of misinformation and nonsense about protein and its role in our diet. For a long time nutritionists and dieticians didn't think protein was a factor in weight control. Then, in the 1970s, high-protein diets became all the rage. They promoted the consumption of all the protein and fat you could eat while eliminating carbohydrates. This type of diet has become all the rage once again, but as we know by now, it's harmful to your health and does nothing to reduce fat cells. High-protein diets have rightly been criticized by nutritionists and doctors alike.

Let's get the facts about protein straight. Proteins are an essential part of your diet. One-half of your dry body weight is made up of protein, i.e., your muscles, organs, skin and hair. Protein is required to build and repair body tissue, and it figures in nearly all metabolic reactions.

Protein is also much more effective than carbohydrates or fat in satisfying hunger. It will make you feel fuller longer, which is why you should always try to incorporate some protein in every meal and snack. It will help keep you alert and feeling full. Again, however, the type of protein you consume is important. Proteins are found in a broad range of food products, both animal and vegetable, and not just in red meat and whole dairy products, which are high in saturated or "bad" fat.

So what sort of protein should you be including in your diet? Choose low-fat proteins: lean or low-fat meats that have been trimmed of any visible fat; skinless poultry; fresh, frozen or canned fish (but not the kind that's coated with batter, which is invariably high in fat); low-fat dairy products like skim milk (believe it or not, after a couple of weeks of drinking it, it tastes just like 2%); low-fat yogurt (look for the artificially sweetened versions, as many manufacturers pump up the sugar as they drop the fat) and low-fat cottage cheese; low-cholesterol liquid eggs; tofu; and soy or whey protein powder, which is great for sprinkling on meals. To most people's surprise the best source of protein may well be the humble bean. Beans are high-protein, low-fat and high-fibre, and they break down slowly in your digestive system, so you feel fuller longer. They can also be added to foods like soups and salads to boost their protein and fibre content. Nuts too are a fine source of protein, with a good monounsaturated fat content. However, because they are so high in fat, you must limit the quantity.

One of the most important things about protein is to spread your daily allowance across all your meals. Too often we grab a hasty breakfast of coffee and toast—a protein-free meal. Lunch is sometimes not much better: a bowl of pasta with steamed vegetables or a green salad with garlic bread. Where's the protein? A typical afternoon snack of a cookie, piece of fruit or muffin contains not a gram of protein. Generally, it's not until dinner that we include protein in our meal, usually our entire daily recommended allowance plus some extra. Because protein is a critical brain food, providing amino acids for the neurotransmitters that relay messages in the brain, it would be better to load up on protein earlier in the day rather than later. That would give you an alert and active mind for your daily activities. However, as I have said, the best solution is to spread your protein consumption throughout the day. This will help keep you on the ball and feeling full.

Now that we know how carbohydrates, fats and proteins work in our digestive system and what makes us gain weight, let's use the science to put together an eating plan that will take off the extra pounds. First, though, let's look at how much weight you should be trying to lose.

TO SUM UP:
1. Include some protein in all your meals and snacks.
2. Eat only low-fat protein, preferably from both animal and vegetable sources.

CHAPTER TWO

How Much Weight Should I Lose?

In this age of excessively and often unhealthily skinny supermodels and TV stars, it's easy to lose sight of what is a healthy weight. Your skin, bones, organs, hair—everything—contribute to your total weight. The only part that you want to reduce is your excess fat, so that's what we have to determine.

There have been many techniques designed to measure excess fat, from measuring pinches of fat (which can be quite misleading) to convoluted formulas and tables requiring higher math. The traditional method, relating weight directly to height through the Metropolitan Life tables, does not tell you how much body fat you're carrying around your waist, hips and thighs, and that's the information you really need to know. So the best method is the Body Mass Index, or BMI. I've included a BMI table on the next page and it's very simple to use. Just find your height in the left vertical column and go across the table until you reach your weight. At the top of that column is your BMI, which is a pretty accurate estimate of the proportion of body fat you're carrying.

BODY MASS INDEX (BMI)

	19	20	21	22	23	24	25	26	27	28	29	30	35	40
Height	**Weight (pounds)**													
4'10"	91	96	100	105	110	115	119	124	129	134	138	143	167	191
4'11"	94	99	104	109	114	119	124	128	133	138	143	148	173	198
5'0"	97	102	107	112	118	123	128	133	138	143	148	153	179	204
5'1"	100	106	111	116	122	127	132	137	143	148	153	158	185	211
5'2"	104	109	115	120	126	131	136	142	147	153	158	164	191	218
5'3"	107	113	118	124	130	135	141	146	152	158	163	169	197	225
5'4"	110	116	122	128	134	140	145	151	157	163	169	174	204	232
5'5"	114	120	126	132	138	144	150	156	162	168	174	180	210	240
5'6"	118	124	130	136	142	148	155	161	167	173	179	186	216	247
5"7"	121	127	134	140	146	153	159	166	172	178	185	191	223	255
5'8"	125	131	138	144	151	158	164	171	177	184	190	197	230	262
5'9"	128	135	142	149	155	162	169	176	182	189	196	203	236	270
5'10"	132	139	146	153	160	167	174	181	188	195	202	207	243	278
5'11"	136	143	150	157	165	172	179	186	193	200	208	215	250	286
6'0"	140	147	154	162	169	177	184	191	199	206	213	221	258	294
6'1"	144	151	159	166	174	182	189	197	204	212	219	227	265	302
6'2"	148	155	163	171	179	186	194	202	210	218	225	233	272	311
6'3"	152	160	168	176	184	192	200	208	216	224	232	240	279	319
6'4"	156	164	172	180	189	197	205	213	221	230	238	246	287	328

Source: U.S. National Heart, Lung and Blood Institute

BMI values less than 18.5 are considered underweight, while those between 25.0 and 29.9 are classified as overweight. BMI values over 30.0 are classified as obese. However, if you are under 5'0", are elderly or overly muscled (and you really have to be a dedicated bodybuilder to qualify), these numbers in all probability do not apply to you.

The ideal BMI for women is between 19 and 24, and for males it's between 20 and 25. These ranges are quite generous, and your target BMI should be toward the lower end of them, say around 22. So put your finger on the BMI number 22 and drop down until you reach your height, which is shown in the left margin. The number at that intersection is what your weight should be to achieve this BMI target.

Let's look at a couple of examples. Mary is 5'6" and weighs 160 pounds. Her BMI is 26, which is 4 notches above her target BMI of 22. This means Mary has to lose 24 pounds in order to bring her to her 22 BMI goal of 136 pounds. Fred is 6'0" and weighs 190 pounds. His BMI is also 26, but he needs to lose 28 pounds to bring his BMI down to the 22 target of 162 pounds.

Another measurement that is important to know is your waist circumference. It indicates your level of abdominal fat, which is significant to your health, especially your heart health. People with a high level of abdominal fat, whom doctors describe as apple-shaped, have a much higher risk of developing cardiovascular disease and Type 2 diabetes (see chapter 9). To measure your waist, take a measuring tape and wrap it around your natural waist just above the navel. Don't be tempted to do a walk-down-the-beach-and-suck-it-in routine. Just stand in a relaxed position and keep the measuring tape from cutting into your flesh. A high-risk waist circumference is thirty-five inches or more for women and forty inches or more for men.

The twenty-four pounds that Mary has to shed and the twenty-eight that Fred needs to lose are pounds of fat—Mary's and Fred's energy storage tanks. In order for them to lose weight they must access and draw down those fat cells. This reminds me of a peculiar contraption used in England during the Second World War. The famous double-decker buses had their upper deck converted into a natural gas tank, consisting of a large fabric balloon. When full, the balloon puffed up several feet above the top of the bus. As it proceeded along its route, the balloon slowly deflated, disappearing by the end of its destination, where it was re-inflated. That's how I visualize our body fat: a deflating balloon from which we draw down our energy, except that in our case the balloon is around our waist, hips and thighs!

So how do you draw down energy from your fat cells? By consuming fewer calories than your body needs. This will force your body to start using its fat stores to make up for the shortfall. Now, I know no one wants to hear about calories, particularly those of us who've tried long and hard to lose weight. Nevertheless, unless you are among those rare and blessed people whose metabolism and genetics enable them to eat as much as they want without gaining an ounce—and if you are, why would you be reading this book?—you, like me and the rest of us mere mortals, are doomed to the inevitable equation. But don't be disheartened: you can easily reduce your daily calorie intake without going hungry and without having to calculate the number of calories in everything you put in your mouth. All you have to do is eat low-G.I. foods (of course!) and adjust the ratio of carbohydrates, fats and proteins in your diet.

Ultimately, all food is a source of energy for our bodies, and we measure energy in calories. The average adult uses somewhere between 1,500 and 3,000 calories a day, depending upon level of activity, rate of metabolism and body weight. What people have been advised to do for decades is to get 55 percent of their calories from carbohydrates, 30 percent from fats and 15 percent from protein. But with our advancing knowledge of nutrition and how our digestive

SOURCE OF CALORIES—THE G.I. DIET

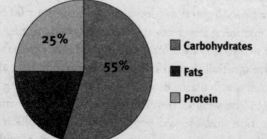

system works, this ratio is being challenged by many physicians and nutritionists. Accordingly, I recommend a modest adjustment to the traditional ratio. You should still get 55 percent of your calories from carbohydrates, but I am recommending that you eat less fat and a bit more protein than what has traditionally been advocated. A recent Harvard School of Public Health study involving over eighty thousand women concluded that a moderately high level of protein intake (24 percent) is beneficial to heart health. Also, the more one exercises, the more protein one needs. Athletes require up to twice the amount of protein as the average person. Though I certainly don't expect you to become an athlete, I will be encouraging more exercise in chapter 8.

Okay, so we now have the ratio that will help us lose those extra pounds. It's all very fine in theory, but what does it mean in the real world? That's what the rest of this book is all about: how much of what to eat, and when. I promised you a simple eating plan that reflects the real world we live in, and that is what I'll give you. The plan is divided into two phases. In Phase I you'll be reducing your caloric intake, burning off those excess fat cells and slimming down to a healthy, ideal weight. This phase takes between three and six months, and it's really a matter of simple math. A pound of fat contains around 3,600 calories. To lose that pound in one week you must reduce your caloric intake by around 500 calories per day (500 x 7 days = 3,500 calories). So if you want to lose twenty pounds, it will take twenty weeks. Here's an example: Mark weighs 180 pounds and he wants to lose 18 pounds. In order to lose a pound a week, Mark must reduce his calorie consumption by 3,500 calories per week. Based on this, it will take Mark 18 weeks to lose 18 pounds. You can look at your own target weight on the chart on the next page to see how long you should expect to be in Phase I of the G.I. Diet.

If twenty-five weeks seems like a long time to you, think of it in terms of the rest of your life. What's half a year compared with the many, many years you'll spend afterwards with a slim, healthy body? This isn't a fad diet—fad diets don't work. The G.I. Diet is a wholesome and surefire route to permanent weight loss.

The reason I've included all this math is to help you understand this diet and how it's going to work for you. But I don't want you to think that you're going to have to do any calculations yourself! They're all built into the program. All you have to do is look at my food guide, which is inserted in the middle of this book and which lists every food that you can think of in one of three categories based on the colours of the stoplight. Foods listed in the red-light or "stop" category are high-G.I., high-fat foods. They include broad beans, melba toast and cheese tortellini, and they should be avoided. These foods are digested so quickly by your body that they are just not worth it. Foods in the yellow-light or "caution" category, for example, muesli, corn and bananas, raise your insulin levels to the point where weight loss is not going to happen, and should therefore be avoided in Phase I as well. The foods that will

TARGET WEIGHT TIMETABLE
(based on 10% weight reduction)

PRESENT WEIGHT	TARGET WEIGHT	WEEKS TO TARGET WEIGHT
120	108	12
130	117	13
140	126	14
150	135	15
160	144	16
170	153	17
180	162	18
190	171	19
200	180	20
210	189	21
220	198	22
230	207	23
240	216	24
250	225	25

make you lose weight are the ones that are listed in the green-light or "go ahead" category. Fettuccine, basmati rice, grapes and many, many others are all green-light foods. Eat them and watch your weight drop.

When you've reached your target BMI, Phase II begins. Here, your calorie input and output are balanced. You're no longer trying to lose weight, so you can start eating foods from the yellow-light category from time to time. All you're doing at this point is maintaining your new weight. Sound simple? It is! So let's get going with Phase I.

TO SUM UP:

1. Set a realistic weight loss target. A BMI of 22 is the ideal goal.

2. In Phase I of the G.I. Diet you'll be reducing the number of calories you consume by adjusting your caloric intake ratio and by eating low-G.I., low-fat foods.

3. When you reach your target BMI, you'll start Phase II of the G.I. Diet, which evens out the number of calories you consume and expend.

CHAPTER THREE

Phase I

Before we go any further, I'd like you to do a little assignment. Try to remember as best you can what you've been eating over the past seven days and fill in the "current" columns of the chart on the next page. This exercise will give you a bit of a reality check and help you to form a baseline or starting point from which you will build your new G.I. Diet program. Later in the book I will ask you to return to this page and record what you've been eating for the past week. I think you'll find the change very interesting—even enlightening.

DAY	BREAKFAST		LUNCH		DINNER		SNACKS	
	CURRENT	G.I. DIET	CURRENT	G.I. DIET	CURRENT	G.I. DIET	CURRENT	G.I. DIET
MONDAY								
TUESDAY								
WEDNESDAY								
THURSDAY								
FRIDAY								
SATURDAY								
SUNDAY								

With the theory and science of the G.I. Diet behind us, it's time to get practical! As you know, Phase I is the weight loss portion of the program, so we'll be sticking with low-G.I., low-fat foods, which we are categorizing as green. In most cases you can eat as much of the green-light foods as you want. It's very important at this stage to eat frequently. This isn't a deprivation diet! So don't leave your digestive system with nothing to do. The saying "The devil finds work for idle hands" also applies to your stomach. If your digestive system is busy processing food and steadily supplying energy to your brain, you won't be looking for high-calorie snacks.

Don't skip breakfast. People who miss breakfast leave their stomachs empty from dinner to lunch the next day—often more than sixteen hours! No wonder they gorge themselves at lunch and then look for a sugar fix mid-afternoon as they run out of steam. Always eat three meals a day—breakfast, lunch and dinner—that contain approximately the same amount of energy (calories), as well as up to three snacks—one mid-morning, one mid-afternoon and one before bed. *Never use sugar.* Instead, use a sugar substitute. And because liquids don't seem to trip our satiety mechanisms, don't waste your calorie allocation on beverages. Always drink water, skim milk and other no-cal or low-cal beverages.

So what can you eat? Let's talk about breakfast first. The following chart lists breakfast foods in the three colour-coded categories. For a comprehensive list, see the colour insert in the middle of this book.

Breakfast

	RED	YELLOW	GREEN
PROTEIN			
Meat and Eggs	Regular bacon	Turkey bacon	Back bacon
	Regular eggs	Whole omega-3 eggs	Lean ham
	Sausages		Low-cholesterol liquid eggs
Dairy	Cheese	Cream cheese (light)	Buttermilk
	Cottage cheese (whole or 2%)	Milk (1%)	Cheese (fat free)
	Cream	Sour cream (light)	Cottage cheese (1% or fat free)
	Milk (whole or 2%)	Yogurt (low fat with sugar)	Fruit yogurt (fat and sugar free)
	Sour cream		Milk (skim)
	Yogurt (whole or 2%)		
CARBOHYDRATES			
Cereals	All cold cereals except those listed as yellow- or green-light	Shredded Wheat Bran	All-Bran
	Granola		Bran Buds
	Muesli (commercial)		Fibre First
			Homemade Muesli (see p. 74)
			Oat bran
			Porridge (large-flake oatmeal)
			Red River

	RED	YELLOW	GREEN
Breads/ Grains	Bagels	Whole grain breads*	100% stone-ground whole wheat*
	Baguette		Apple Bran Muffins (see p. 89)
	Cookies		Homemade Granola Bars (see p. 90)
	Croissants		Whole-grain, high-fibre breads (2½–3 g fibre per slice)*
	Donuts		
	Muffins		
	Pancakes/Waffles		
	White bread		
Fruits	Applesauce containing sugar	Apricots (fresh and dried)	Apples
	Canned fruit in syrup	Bananas	Berries
	Melons	Fruit cocktail in juice	Cherries
	Most dried fruit	Kiwi	Grapefruit
		Mango	Grapes
		Papaya	Oranges
		Pineapple	Peaches
			Plums
Juices	Fruit drinks	Apple (unsweetened)	Eat the fruit rather than drink its juice
	Prune	Grapefruit (unsweetened)	
	Sweetened juices	Orange (unsweetened)	
	Watermelon	Pear (unsweetened)	

* Use a single slice only per serving.

	RED	YELLOW	GREEN
Vegetables	French fries		Most vegetables*
	Hash browns		
FATS			
	Butter	Most nuts	Almonds**
	Hard margarine	Soft margarine (non-hydrogenated)	Canola oil**
	Tropical oils	Vegetable oils	Hazelnuts**
	Vegetable shortening		Olive oil**
			Soft margarine (non-hydrogenated, light)**

* See colour insert for complete list.
** Use sparingly.

Juice

- Always eat the fruit or vegetable rather than drink its juice. Juice is a processed product that is more rapidly digested than the parent fruit. To illustrate the point: diabetics who run into an insulin crisis and are in a state of hypoglycemia (low blood sugar) are usually given orange juice, which is the fastest way to get glucose into the bloodstream. A glass of juice has 2 1/2 times the calories of a fresh whole orange.

Cereals

- Large-flake or slow-cooking porridge oats are the best choice for two reasons: oatmeal stays with you all morning, and it's great for your heart as it lowers cholesterol. (The cooking time is only around three minutes in the microwave.) Oat bran is also excellent.

- Among cold cereals, go for the high-fibre products—the ones that have at least 10 grams of fibre per serving. Fibre content is clearly indicated on cereal packages. Cereal manufacturers, to their credit, were among the first to voluntarily publish nutritional facts.

- High-fibre cereals are a great base to which fruit, nuts and yogurt may be added.

Dairy

- The beverage of choice is skim milk. I had a real problem with skim milk both on cereal and as a beverage, but I persevered. Move down from 2% to 1% to skim in stages. I find that 2% tastes like cream now!

- Yogurt is a real plus. But look for low- or no-fat versions and, just as important, look for the artificially sweetened products. (Aspartame is the most commonly used artificial sweetener.) Regular low-fat yogurts have nearly twice the calories as the aspartame versions. (There has been a considerable amount of negative publicity, generated principally by the sugar industry, about artificial sweeteners. This has triggered dozens of studies worldwide, none of which have shown any long-term risks to our health. These products are safe and of real value in calorie control. But, as with most foods, don't go overboard.)

- Cottage cheese is an excellent and filling source of protein. Again, go for the 1% or fat-free variety. Add fruit or light fruit spreads for flavour.

- Use other dairy products sparingly. Avoid most cheeses like the plague; their high saturated fat heads straight for your arteries. The dairy industry has a lot to answer for when it comes to our health. The success of their massive cheese advertising and promotion campaigns, often aimed at children, is reprehensible. If cheese is your thing, then go for the no-fat options or use stronger-flavoured ones, such as Stilton or feta, sprinkled sparingly as a flavour enhancer.

Bread

- Always use 100-percent stone-ground whole wheat, or any other whole-grain bread that has 2 1/2 to 3 grams of fibre per slice. "Stone ground" is important because stones grind grain more coarsely than the steel rollers that grind most of our flour. The coarser the grind, the less the fibre is separated, resulting in a far lower G.I.

Eggs

- Choose low-cholesterol, low-fat eggs in liquid form (250 ml carton = 5 eggs). Unlike regular eggs, which are high in cholesterol, eggs in liquid form are a great green-light product. Go for them.

Spreads

- Do not use butter. The latest premium brands of non-hydrogenated soft margarine are acceptable and the light versions even more so.

- In fruit spreads look for the "double fruit no added sugar" versions. These taste terrific and are remarkably low in calories.

Bacon

- Sorry, but regular bacon is a red-light food. Acceptable alternatives are Canadian back bacon, turkey bacon and lean ham.

Coffee

- Coffee ideally should be decaffeinated (see page 61). Never add sugar and use only 1% or skim milk.

Lunch

Because lunch is the meal most of us eat outside the home, it can be the most problematic, limited by time, budget and availability considerations. There are, however, some practical guidelines.

		RED	YELLOW	GREEN
PROTEIN				
Meat, Poultry, Fish and Eggs		Ground beef (more than 10% fat)	Ground beef (lean)	All fish and seafood, fresh or frozen (no batter or breading) or canned
		Hamburgers	Lamb (lean cuts)	Beef (lean cuts)
		Hot dogs	Pork (lean cuts)	Chicken breast (skinless)
		Processed meats	Turkey bacon	Ground beef (extra-lean)
		Regular bacon	Whole omega-3 eggs	Lean deli ham
		Sausages		Low-cholesterol liquid eggs
		Whole regular eggs		Turkey breast (skinless)
				Veal
Dairy		Cheese	Milk (1%)	Cheese (fat free)
		Cottage cheese (whole or 2%)	Cheese (low fat)	Cottage cheese (1% or fat free)
		Cream cheese	Yogurt (low fat with sugar)	Fruit yogurt (fat and sugar free)
		Milk (whole or 2%)	Cream cheese (light)	Ice cream (low fat and no added sugar)
				Milk (skim)

	RED	YELLOW	GREEN
CARBOHYDRATES			
Breads/ Grains	Bagels	Whole grain breads*	100% stone-ground whole wheat*
	Baguette/ Croissants		Pasta* (fettuccine, spaghetti, penne, vermicelli, linguine, macaroni)
	Cake/Cookies		Rice (basmati, wild, brown, long grain)
	Hamburger Buns		Whole-grain, high-fibre breads (2½–3 g fibre per slice)*
	Macaroni and cheese		
	Muffins/Donuts		
	Noodles (canned or instant)		
	Pancakes/Waffles		
	Pasta filled with cheese or meat		
	Pizza		
	Rice (short grain, white, instant)		

	RED	YELLOW	GREEN	
Fruits/ Vegeta- bles	Broad beans	Apricots	Apples	Lettuce
	French fries	Bananas	Asparagus	Mushrooms
	Melons	Corn	Avocado	Olives*
	Most dried fruit	Kiwi	Beans (green/wax)	Onions
	Potatoes (mashed or baked)	Papaya	Bell peppers	Oranges (all varieties)

* Limit serving size.

RED	YELLOW	GREEN	
	Pineapple	Blackberries	Peaches
	Potatoes (boiled)	Broccoli	Pears
		Brussels sprouts	Peas
		Cabbage	Peppers (hot)
		Carrots	Pickles
		Cauliflower	Plums
		Celery	Potatoes (boiled new)
		Cherries	Radishes
		Cucumbers	Raspberries
		Eggplant	Snow peas
		Grapefruit	Spinach
		Grapes	Strawberries
		Leeks	Tomatoes
		Lemons	Zucchini
RED	YELLOW	GREEN	

FATS

RED	YELLOW	GREEN
Butter	Mayonnaise (light)	Almonds*
Hard margarine	Most nuts	Canola oil*
Mayonnaise	Salad dressings (light)	Mayonnaise (fat free)
Salad dressings (regular)	Soft margarine (non-hydrogenated)	Olive oil*
Tropical oils		Salad dressings (fat free)
Vegetable shortening		Soft margarine (non-hydrogenated, light)

* Use sparingly.

RED	YELLOW	GREEN
SOUPS		
All cream-based soups	Chicken noodle	Chunky bean and vegetable soups
Black bean	Lentil	(e.g., Campbell's
Green pea	Tomato	Healthy Request,
Puréed vegetable		Healthy Choice and
Split pea		Too Good To Be True)

Bread

- Sandwiches are probably the most popular choice for lunch in North America, and they usually have a high G.I. and are high in calories. But you don't have to cut sandwiches out of your diet. To lower their impact on your hips, choose sandwiches made with whole wheat or whole grain bread, the grittier the better. Then take off the top layer of the bread and eat the sandwich open-faced. Watch out for mayonnaise—it's often hidden in egg, chicken and tuna salad. Always ask for no mayo—unless it's non- or low fat. Also request no butter or margarine on bread. Hummus or mustard are good alternatives. Sorry, but peanut butter, even the "lite" version, is red-light. Though it is low G.I., it is incredibly calorie-dense.

Fast Food

- The simple answer to "Should I visit fast-food outlets for lunch?" is NO. With a few exceptions, fast food is loaded with saturated fat and calories, with rarely a gram of fibre in sight. For example, a Quarter Pounder with cheese hits you with just under 500 calories and over half your day's quota of fat. Even the carrot muffin comes loaded with similar calories and fat. Merely being in the presence of all those tempting burgers, fries and shakes makes your challenges more difficult—so stay away if at all possible! I can assure you that after a few months on the G.I. Diet, even the idea of fast food will turn you off. With your face pressed to the window of McDonald's, you'll watch with amazement what the heavyweights are putting away—straight to their waists and hips. That could have been you!

    If your alternatives are limited, here is how you can sucessfully navigate through this gastronomic minefield.

Burgers: Dispose of the top of the bun and don't order cheese or bacon. Keep it as simple as possible.

Fries: DON'T. A medium order of McDonald's fries contains 17 grams of fat (mostly saturated), about 50 percent of your total daily allowance.

Milkshakes: DON'T. The saturated fat and calorie levels are unbelievable.

Salads: Go for them, as much as you like, but beware the red flashing light over most dressings. Always use light or low-fat dressings as they have less than a third of the calories of regular dressings. Failing that, use oil and vinegar. Ask for your dressing on the side so you can control the quantity. Avoid Caesar salads as their high-fat dressing can be disastrous.

Wraps: An increasingly popular alternative to the traditional sandwich is a wrap. Ask if the pita bread can be split in half. (My lunch counter thinks I'm odd in this regard and insists on giving me the other half in a separate bag to take with me. I've no idea what they expect me to do with it!)

Submarines: Ask for a whole wheat roll but again, eat it open-faced. Avoid cheese and mayo unless they're low-fat.

Fish: An excellent choice providing there's no batter or breaded coating.

Chinese: The two things to watch for are the rice and the sauces, especially the sweet ones, which are high in sugar. Rice is usually a problem, as most restaurants use a glutinous high-G.I. rice whose grains tend to stick together. If you can be assured the rice is either basmati or long grain and doesn't clump together, then okay, but limit the quantity to a quarter of your plate.

Pasta

- Though most pastas range in the moderate G.I. category, some are clearly preferable to others. A rule of thumb is that thicker pastas are better. Pasta is a villain in our obesity problem not because of any issue with pasta itself— a moderate-G.I. and low-fat (although high-calorie) product—but due to the quantities we eat. Italians are aghast at the huge bowls of pasta we consume as our main course. They quite correctly view pasta as an appetizer or a side dish. We typically view it as the bulk of the meal, with sauce and a few pieces of protein on top.

  Because it's difficult when dining out to order a partial plate of pasta, it's best to avoid it completely. If you are able to obtain a side order, then limit the quantity to cover a quarter of the plate (about 3/4 cup) and ask for low-fat sauce options. Please, no alfredo. Whole grain pasta is by far your best choice.

Soups

- A chunky bean or vegetable soup followed by fish or chicken makes an ideal lunch. Beware of cream-based or puréed vegetable soups; they are high in fat and heavily processed, therefore red light all the way.

Potatoes

- Since it's almost impossible to get plain, boiled new potatoes (see page 52) when eating out, always ask your waiter for double vegetables in lieu of potatoes. In two years, after dozens of requests, I've never been refused.

Rice

- Eat basmati, brown, wild or long-grain rice only, and in quantities to cover no more than a quarter of your plate. Avoid rice if it's glutinous and sticky.

Dessert

- Fat- and sugar-free yogurt is a terrific choice. Always eat some fruit. I keep a supply of apples, pears, peaches and grapes, depending on the season, in my office. Stay away from most other desserts.

Snacks

Because it's a bad idea to leave your stomach empty, snacks are an important part of the G.I. Diet. But I'm afraid you'll have to avoid the customary choices like muffins, cookies and chips, all high-G.I. foods that are calorie-dense. Two hours after eating them you've added a few more fat cells and are feeling hungry again. These foods are just not worth the trouble!

Phase I snacks include fruit, fat- and sugar-free yogurt, 1% cottage cheese and raw vegetables. You might also want to explore the world of food bars. Stay away from the expensive high-carbohydrate, high-calorie sugar bars, choosing instead those that have a more balanced ratio of carbohydrates, fats and proteins. Half a Balance Bar or Power Bar is an excellent snack, and so are most bars that weigh between 50 and 65 grams and have around 200 calories. They should contain 20 to 30 grams of carbohydrates, 12 to 15 grams of protein and only 5 grams of fat. Check labels carefully.

If you bake your own low-G.I. muffins and granola bars (the recipes are in chapter 5), they also make good snacks. You can freeze a batch or two and reheat them in the microwave.

RED	YELLOW	GREEN
Candy	Bananas	Almonds*
Cookies	Dark chocolate (60–70% cocoa)	Apple Bran Muffins (see p. 89)
Crackers	Most nuts*	Applesauce (unsweetened)
Donuts	Popcorn (light, microwaveable)	Canned peaches or pears in juice or water
Ice cream		Cottage cheese (1% or fat free)
Muffins (commercial)		Food bars**
Popcorn (regular)		Fruit yogurt (fat and sugar free)
Potato chips		Hazelnuts*
Pretzels		Homemade Granola Bars (see p. 90)
Raisins		Ice cream (low fat, no added sugar)
Rice cakes		Most fresh fruit
Tortilla chips		Most fresh vegetables
Trail mix		

* Limit serving.

** *Warning:* Most so-called nutrition bars are high-G.I. and high-calorie, with a lot of quick-fix carbs. Look for 50–65 g bars, around 200 calories, with 20–30 g carbohydrates, 12–15 g protein and 5 g fat per bar.

Dinner

Dinner, traditionally, is the main meal of the day—and the one where most of us blow our diet to shreds. Unlike breakfast and lunch, dinner doesn't usually have any time or availability constraints (although juggling our schedules along with our children's can sometimes make this a moot point).

The typical North American dinner comprises three things: meat or fish; potato, pasta or rice; and vegetables. Together, these foods provide an assortment of carbohydrates, proteins and fats, along with other minerals and vitamins essential to our health.

	RED	YELLOW	GREEN
PROTEIN			
Meat, Poultry, Fish and Eggs	Ground beef (more than 10% fat)	Ground beef (lean)	All fish and seafood
	Hamburgers	Lamb (lean cuts)	Beef (lean cuts)
	Hot dogs	Pork (lean cuts)	Chicken breast (skinless)
	Processed meats	Whole omega-3 eggs	Ground beef (extra lean)
	Sausages		Lean deli ham
	Whole regular eggs		Low-cholesterol liquid eggs
			Turkey breast (skinless)
			Veal
Dairy	Cheese	Cheese (low fat)	Cheese (fat free)

	RED	YELLOW	GREEN
	Cottage cheese (whole or 2%)	Milk (1%)	Cottage cheese (1% or fat free)
	Milk (whole or 2%)	Sour cream (light)	Fruit yogurt (fat and sugar free)
	Sour cream	Yogurt (low fat)	Milk (skim)
	Yogurt (whole or 2%)		

CARBOHYDRATES

	RED	YELLOW	GREEN
Breads/ Grains	Bagels	Whole grain breads*	100% stone-ground whole wheat*
	Baguette/Croissants		Pasta* (fettuccine, spaghetti, penne, vermicelli, linguine, macaroni)
	Cake/Cookies		
	Macaroni & cheese		
	Muffins/Donuts		
	Noodles (canned or instant)		Rice* (basmati, wild, brown, long grain)
	Pasta filled with cheese or meat		Whole-grain, high-fibre breads (2½–3 g fibre per slice)
	Pizza		
	Rice (short grain white, instant)		
	Tortillas		

	RED	YELLOW	GREEN	
Fruits/ Vegeta- bles	Broad beans	Apricots	Apples	Lettuce
	French fries	Bananas	Asparagus	Mushrooms
	Melons	Corn	Avocado	Olives*
	Most dried fruit	Kiwi	Beans (green/wax)	Onions

* Limit serving size.

RED	YELLOW	GREEN	
Potatoes (mashed or baked)	Papaya	Bell peppers	Oranges (all varieties)
	Pineapple	Blackberries	Peaches
	Potatoes (boiled)	Broccoli	Pears
		Brussels sprouts	Peas
		Cabbage	Peppers (hot)
		Carrots	Pickles
		Cauliflower	Plums
		Celery	Potatoes (boiled new)
		Cherries	Radishes
		Cucumbers	Raspberries
		Eggplant	Snow peas
		Grapefruit	Spinach
		Grapes	Strawberries
		Leeks	Tomatoes
		Lemons	Zucchini
RED	YELLOW	GREEN	

FATS

RED	YELLOW	GREEN
Butter	Mayonnaise (light)	Almonds*
Hard margarine	Salad dressings (light)	Canola oil*
Mayonnaise	Soft margarine (non-hydrogenated)	Hazelnuts*
Salad dressings (regular)		Mayonnaise (fat free)

* Use sparingly.

RED	YELLOW	GREEN
Tropical oils		Olive oil*
Vegetable shortening		Salad dressings (fat free)
		Soft margarine (non-hydrogenated, light)

SOUPS

RED	YELLOW	GREEN
All cream-based soups	Chicken noodle	Chunky bean and vegetable soups
Black bean	Lentil	(e.g., Campbell's
Green pea	Tomato	Healthy Request,
Puréed vegetable		Healthy Choice and
Split pea		Too Good To Be True)

* Use sparingly.

Meat/Fish

- Most meats contain saturated (bad) fat, so it's important to buy lean cuts or trim off all the visible fat. A loin steak trimmed to only a quarter-inch of fat can have up to twice the fat of a steak with no trim. Obviously, some cuts of meat have intrinsically higher fat content. Check with your butcher if in doubt.

- Chicken or turkey are excellent choices *provided all the skin is removed.*

- Fish and seafood are also excellent choices. Though certain fish, such as salmon, have a relatively high oil content, this oil is extremely beneficial to your health, especially heart health.

- In terms of quantity, the best measure for meat or fish is your palm. The portion should fit into the palm of your hand and be about as thick. Another good visual is a pack of cards—so my friends with small palms tell me!

Potatoes

- Potatoes' G.I. ranges from moderate to high, depending on the type and how they are cooked and served. In the lowest G.I. category are boiled new potatoes served whole or sliced, two to three per serving. (The G.I. for boiled new potatoes is 56, while baked have a G.I. of 84.) All other versions are strictly red light.

Pasta

- Thicker pastas generally have a lower G.I., but as mentioned earlier, the serving size is critical. Pasta should be a side dish and not form the base of the meal. In other words, it should take up only a quarter of your plate. Whole wheat pasta, available at most natural food stores and increasingly in your local supermarket, is preferable. Allow 35 grams of dried pasta per serving or 3/4 cup cooked.

Rice

- Rice has a broad G.I. range. The best choices are basmati, wild, brown or long-grain. These rices contain a starch, amylose, that breaks down more slowly than other rices. Again, serving size is critical. Allow three tablespoons of dry rice per serving, or 2/3 cup cooked.

Vegetables/Salad

- This is where you can go wild. Eat as many vegetables and as much salad as you like. In fact, this should be the backbone of your meal. Virtually all vegetables are ideal. Try to have a side salad with your daily dinner.

- Watch out for salad dressings. Use only low-fat and fat-free ones.

- Serve two or three varieties of vegetables for dinner. Frozen bags of mixed, unseasoned vegetables are inexpensive and convenient.

Desserts

- This is one of the most troublesome issues in any weight control program. Desserts usually taste great, but they tend to be loaded with sugar and fat—a real guilt-inducing situation! As the last course in most meals, desserts often fall into the "Should I or shouldn't I?" category.

  The good news is that dessert should be a part of your meal. There are a broad range of low-G.I., low-calorie alternatives that taste great and are good for you. Virtually any fruit qualifies (though hold off on the bananas and raisins) and there are numerous fat- and sugar-free dairy products such as yogurt and ice cream. You won't be eating apple pie à la mode, but you could be enjoying applesauce with yogurt, or even a meringue with fresh or frozen berries.

As a basis for comparison, you may be interested to know what the typical Canadian diet currently looks like:

Vegetables: Too few are consumed, but among the most popular are potatoes, carrots, lettuce (iceberg), tomatoes, corn and onions.

Rice (mainly plain white): Eaten once a week in 50 percent of households, but more often in larger families.

Pasta: Eighty percent eat pasta on a weekly basis. Older people eat less. Americans, interestingly enough, consume one-third more than Canadians.

Poultry/Meat/Fish: Top spot goes to beef and chicken, closely followed by pork. Fish is eaten once a week by 50 percent of households, and three-quarters of these servings have batter or breading.

Soup: Sixty-five percent of us have soup at least once a week, with broth-based soups being more popular than cream. Hurray!

Cheese: Eighty-five percent consume at least one serving a week.

Eggs: Sixty-five percent eat eggs at least once a week.

Portions

Understanding portions is essential if the G.I. Diet is to work for you. Since most vegetables and fruits have a low G.I. rating and are low in calories and fat, they are the most important food group in the G.I. Diet. However, both the Canadian and U.S. governments suggest that grains should be the most important food group. If you look at the United States Department of Agriculture's Food Pyramid on the next page, you will see that it suggests grains should be the largest component of your diet, followed by vegetables and fruit. But by giving grains priority, governments and most nutritionists are promoting the leading cause of overweight and obesity. The Mayo Clinic has recently changed its Healthy Weight Pyramid to promote vegetables and fruits as the base of a healthy diet, rather than grains, and this is exactly what the G.I. Diet recommends. (See the G.I. Diet Food Pyramid on page 57.)

USDA FOOD PYRAMID

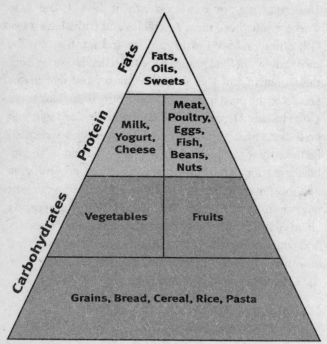

Source: U.S. Department of Agriculture

THE G.I. FOOD PYRAMID

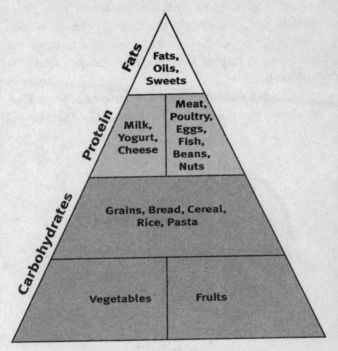

To translate the pyramid to your dinner plate, dish out enough vegetables to cover 50 percent of your plate, enough meat, poultry or fish to cover 25 percent of your plate, and enough rice, pasta or potatoes to cover the remaining 25 percent. Don't bend the rules by piling your food too high!

Below is a diagram of the way we traditionally visualize our dinner plate followed by the healthier G.I. Diet version.

TRADITIONAL

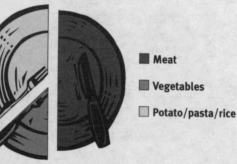

■ Meat

■ Vegetables

□ Potato/pasta/rice

G.I. DIET

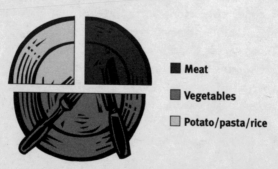

■ Meat

■ Vegetables

□ Potato/pasta/rice

Vegetarians

Most people I know who are vegetarian don't need to lose weight. My middle son is a vegetarian, and at six foot five and 160 pounds he looks undernourished. But if you are a non–meat eater and need to lose weight, the G.I. Diet is the program for you. All you have to do is continue to substitute vegetable protein for animal protein—something you've been doing all along. However, because most vegetable protein sources, such as beans, are encased in fibre, your digestive system may not be getting the maximum protein benefit. So try to add easily digestible protein boosters like tofu and soy protein powder.

Beverages

Since 70 percent of our body is made up of water, it's hardly surprising that drinking fluids is an important part of any dietary program. Most dieticians recommend eight glasses of fluid per day. This sounds a bit steep to me, and every time I make a conscious effort to comply I find myself running for the bathroom every couple of hours!

If you set out to drink eight glasses, in reality you end up consuming a great deal more than that. The reason is that we take in a great deal of fluid without being conscious of it. Add together other liquids you consume such as milk in cereal, and soft drinks, along with the water that makes up a great deal of the bulk of most fruits and vegetables, and you easily end up taking in several cups a day without even trying. *So the rule of thumb is: drink at least a glass of water with each of your three main meals and with each snack.*

Now, what to drink?

Water

The cheapest and best choice is plain, simple water. Try to drink an eight-ounce glass of water *before* each meal and snack, for two reasons. First, having your stomach partly filled with liquid before the meal means you will feel full more quickly, thus reducing the temptation to overeat. Second, you won't be tempted to "wash down" your food before it's been sufficiently chewed, thus upsetting your digestive system.

Soft Drinks

If water is too boring for you, go for sugar-free soft drinks, preferably also caffeine-free (see Coffee, on the next page). Remember, the sugar in a drink is less satisfying than an equal quantity of sugar in food, so don't waste your calorie intake quota.

Skim Milk

My personal preference of beverage is skim milk, at least with breakfast and lunch. It's an ideal green-light food, and since most lunches tend to be protein deficient, drinking skim milk is a good way of making up some of the shortfall.

Coffee

The principal problem with coffee is caffeine. Caffeine stimulates gastric juices, which in turn stimulate appetite. So try to curb your caffeine intake by limiting yourself to a cup of coffee per day. An alternative is decaffeinated coffee—no hardship given the delicious range of decaffeinated options available today.

As an experiment I asked a group of dinner guests whether they preferred caffeinated or decaffeinated coffee. It split about fifty-fifty. I then served decaffeinated coffee (a plug for Starbucks here) to everyone and asked how they liked it. I received more applause from those who had asked for caffeinated than from the dedicated decaf aficionados! I rest my case.

Tea

Tea has considerably less caffeine than coffee. Both black and green teas also contain an antioxidant property that appears to carry a significant heart health benefit. In fact there are higher quantities of flavonoids (antioxidants) in tea than in any vegetable tested. Two cups of tea have the same amount of antioxidants as seven cups of orange juice or twenty of apple juice. Maybe my ninety-three-year-old mother and her tea-drinking cronies are on to something.

So, tea in moderation is fine. If you are looking for alternative teas that are completely caffeine-free, there has been an explosion of flavoured herbal and fruit options, though they don't have the antioxidant characteristics of real tea. In fact, as I'm writing this, I'm drinking English Toffee tea—delicious! These teas are a lot of fun and taste great.

Fruit Drinks/Juices

Fruit drinks contain a large amount of sugar, are calorie-dense and definitely belong on the red-light list.

Fruit juices are preferable, but as we discussed earlier, it is always better to eat the fruit or vegetable rather than drink its juice. Remember, the more work your body has to do to break down food, the better. There is nothing worse than an idle stomach!

Alcohol

I'm sure this is the section that most readers fast-forwarded to. Well, it's a good news, bad news story.

The good news is that alcohol in moderation (and we'll discuss moderation in chapter 7) is not only acceptable but, as you'll learn later, can even be good for your health.

The bad news is that alcohol in general is a disaster for weight control. Alcohol is easily metabolized by the body, which means increased insulin production, a drop in blood sugar levels, and demand from the body for more alcohol or food to boost those sagging sugar levels. This is a vicious circle that can play havoc with your weight loss plans. To make things worse, most alcoholic drinks are loaded with empty calories.

So, NO ALCOHOL at all in Phase I.

Serving Size

Some nutritionists contend that today's weight problems are as much to do with serving size as with the
type of food we eat. There is a great deal of truth to this.
The "Big Mac" mentality has permeated our thinking.
If one serving tastes terrific, think what two can do!

A trip to the movies encapsulates the problem. All
popcorn, drinks and candy come in giant sizes only. The
fast-food industry in particular has recognized our
desire to treat ourselves when we eat out by ordering
larger servings, and they do everything to encourage
that tendency. Food is a relatively cheap commodity,
especially when it is high in low-cost simple carbohydrates such as sugar and flour. That is why fast-food
companies can offer bigger servings at very little incre-
mental cost.

The golden rule is *moderation*. Earlier we showed a way
of looking at your plate to assess portion sizes. All fruits
and vegetables in the green-light section can be eaten in
virtually unlimited quantities. That's why they make great
snack foods. The recommended serving size for meat and
fish is 4 ounces, for pasta it's 3/4 cup cooked, and for rice
it's 2/3 cup cooked. Many packaged foods indicate serving
size and this is usually a reliable guideline as they tend to
be conservative (usually so that the calorie or fat levels
appear lower).

As in most things, common sense should be your
guide. This book promised to keep things simple and not

have you counting calories or using other complex ways to measure food. If anything is going to turn you off a weight-loss program, it would be difficult formulas, weights and measures. Accordingly, most serving sizes recommended in this book are an average. There is some latitude on either side, depending on how your body weight varies from the broad average—125 to 150 pounds for women and 140 to 175 for men. Adjust serving sizes down if you fall below the average, up if you are over. But to make it work and keep things simple, you have to do your part by using your own judgment. As with juries and democracy, the common sense of the public should not be underestimated!

TO SUM UP:

1. In Phase I eat exclusively green-light foods, i.e., those with a low glycemic and calorie rating.
2. Eat three principal meals of equal nutritional value per day plus three between-meal snacks.
3. Drink lots of water or diet soft drinks, including an eight-ounce glass before or with each meal and snack. And don't touch caffeine or alcohol until Phase II!
4. Moderation and common sense are your guides for determining serving portions.

CHAPTER FOUR

Ready, Set, Go!

Ready

By now, I hope you understand the principles of the G.I. Diet and are totally convinced that the plan is going to work for you (and your family) for the rest of your life. All that's left is to take the plunge. This is what I call the READY stage, and it is perhaps the most agonizing part of the journey.

The best advice I can give comes from my own experience. I knew I had to lose twenty pounds to take me to the 22 BMI target weight. On the advice of a friend I gathered together a number of books (diet books!) and piled them on my bathroom scale until they totalled twenty pounds. I then put them in a backpack and carried them around the house one Sunday morning. By noon the weight was really bugging me. What a relief it was to take the bag off my back! So the question was, did I want to carry that excess twenty pounds of fat around with me each and every day, or lose it and gain the sense of lightness and freedom I experienced after the backpack came off?

I urge you to try the same exercise. Identify how much weight you want to lose by using the BMI chart on page 21. Bundle up a sufficient number of books to equal that weight and carry them on your back or shoulder, or around your waist, for a few hours. Remember, that's the excess weight you are permanently carrying around with you. No wonder you feel exhausted! And that's one of the principal benefits of the G.I. Diet: not only will you look and feel great, but you will rediscover all that energy and zip you had in your teens and twenties, which you thought had been lost forever.

SET

Wondering what to do first? Well, let me suggest that you proceed in the following manner:

1. Baseline

Before you do anything else, get your vital statistics on record. Measuring progress is a great motivator. You will find a detachable log sheet on page 155 to keep in the bathroom and record your weekly progress. There are two key measurements. The first is weight. Always weigh yourself at the same time of day, because a meal or bowel movement can throw out your weight by a couple of pounds. First thing in the morning, before you eat breakfast, is a good time. The other important measurement is your waist. Measure at your natural waistline—usually just above the navel while standing in a relaxed, normal posture. The tape should be snug but not indenting the skin.

Record both measurements on the bathroom log. I've added a Comments column to the log sheet where you can note how you're feeling, or any unusual events in the past week that might have some bearing on your progress.

2. Pantry

Clear out your pantry, fridge and freezer of all red- and yellow-light products. Give them to a food bank or your neighbours. If the products aren't around, you won't be tempted to eat or drink them.

3. Shopping

Stock up at home on products that get a green light. There is a Green-Light Pantry Guide on page 131, and if you turn to page 135 you will find a detachable shopping list to take with you to the grocery store. There are a few yellow-light products that have been asterisked, and these can be used sparingly during your Phase I weight loss period. After a couple of trips, selecting the right products will become second nature.

Although we've tried to provide a broad range of products, we could not hope to cover all the thousands of brands available in most supermarkets. This means you have to check labels when in doubt. In general, if a manufacturer has not put content information on the label, avoid its products; it probably has something to hide.

For products or brands we do not list, look for three things:

1. Calorie content per serving. Note: check that the serving size is realistic.

2. Fat level, especially of saturated fat or trans fatty acids (usually called hydrogenated). Look for a minimum ratio of 3 grams of poly- or monounsaturated fat to each gram of saturated fat. Keep total fat to less than 10 grams per serving.

3. Fibre level. Remember, fibrous foods have a lower G.I. Look for a minimum of 4 to 5 grams of fibre per serving.

Basically, we're shopping for foods that are low-calorie, low-fat (especially saturated) and high-fibre. That's the formula for all our green-light products: they have a low G.I. and are calorie-light. By eating these foods we reduce our calorie intake without going hungry.

You will be buying considerably more fruit and vegetables than previously, so be a little daring and try some varieties that are new to you. There's a wonderful world of fresh and frozen produce just waiting for you to enjoy!

Caution: Don't go food shopping with an empty stomach or you'll end up buying items that don't belong on the G.I. Diet!

GO

Now that the difficult part is done, it's plain sailing from here. Don't be surprised if you lose more than one pound per week in the first few weeks, as your body adjusts to the new regimen. Most of that weight will be water, not fat. Remember, 70 percent of our body weight is water.

Don't worry if from time to time you "fall off the wagon," eating or drinking with friends and going outside the program. That's the real world, and though it will marginally delay your target date, it's more important that you not feel as though you're living in a straitjacket. I probably live about 90 percent within the program and 10 percent outside—by choice. The fact is, I feel better and more energized when on the program and rarely feel deprived. However, in Phase I, try to keep these lapses to a minimum; you will be able to allow yourself more leeway once you have achieved your target weight.

If you want further proof or reassurance that your new way of eating is really working, try this test. After eight weeks on the G.I. Diet, break all the rules and have a lunch consisting of a whole pizza with the works, a bread roll and a beer or regular soft drink. While you're at it, finish up with a slice of pie. I'll spare you the ice cream.

I did just that, and by about three in the afternoon I could hardly keep awake. I felt listless and worn out. I hadn't planned on eating so much but got caught up in a fellow employee's farewell lunch. The reason for my afternoon fatigue (which you've likely figured out for yourself) was the combination of high-G.I. foods (pizza, bread roll, beer and pie), which led to a rapid spike in my blood sugar level. The resulting rush of insulin drained this sugar from my blood and caused my sugar levels to drop precipitously, leaving my brain and muscles starved of energy, i.e., in a hypoglycemic state. No wonder I couldn't keep my eyes open.

Here are some tips to keep you motivated, especially when your resolve starts flagging (as it inevitably will from time to time):

1. Maintain a weekly progress log. (A removable log sheet appears on page 155.) Nothing is more motivating than success.

2. Set up a reward system. Buy yourself a small gift when you achieve a predetermined weight goal—perhaps a gift for every three pounds lost.

3. Identify family members or friends who will be your cheerleaders. Make them active participants in your plan. Even better, find a friend who will join the plan for mutual support.

4. Avoid acquaintances and haunts that may encourage your old behaviours. You know who I mean!

5. Try adding what my friend calls a special "spa" day to your week—a day when you are *especially good* with your program. This gives you some extra credit in your weight loss account to draw on when the inevitable relapse occurs.

6. Sign up for the free G.I. Diet newsletter to learn from readers' experiences and keep up to date on the latest developments in diet and health (details on **www.gidiet.com**).

TO SUM UP:
1. Try the weighted backpack test.
2. Take baseline weight and waist measurements.
3. Clear the pantry, fridge and freezer of all red- and yellow-light products.
4. Shop for green-light products to restock your pantry, fridge and freezer.
5. Follow the five tips above this box, and do keep a record of your progress.
6. *Go for it!*

CHAPTER FIVE

Meal Ideas

When I wrote the first draft of this book, I neglected to include any recipes. My wife read the manuscript and suggested that readers would find some recipes useful, especially when getting started. Since following the G.I. Diet requires us to change how we normally eat, she felt that including recipes would demonstrate how you might adapt your own favourites to make them green-light. She suggested that my lack of enthusiasm for including recipes had more to do with my own culinary incompetence (quite true) than with any pedagogical stratagems.

So, stung to action and under her direction, I am offering suggestions for the three primary meals and snacks for Phase I of the G.I. Diet. I have tried to adapt meals that are commonly used by most of us, so there is no need to worry about the unfamiliar. In these recipes I have not only used green-light foods, but I've also kept the use of fats in cooking down to a minimum. Always use non-stick pans, since they allow you to use only a small amount of fat when cooking. Use either a teaspoon or two of canola or olive oil, or even better, use a vegetable oil spray.

Remember, there are 2,000 calories in one cup of oil. Grilling or barbecuing are excellent ways of cooking meat, since the fat from the meat drops into the pan or onto the coals.

Cutting fat doesn't mean you have to cut flavour or lose that all-important taste sensation. Cream can be replaced by yogurt, yogurt cheese (see page 87) or cottage cheese. Use fat-free mayonnaise in tuna or chicken salads. You can still use cheese, especially the strongly flavoured ones, *but sprinkle it sparingly as a flavour enhancer only*, rather than using it as the prime ingredient. Try some new spices and flavoured vinegars. Salsa will spice up many foods without adding calories or fat, and ginger adds life to stir-fries.

Breakfast

Oatmeal is the king of breakfast foods—low-G.I. and low-calorie, easy to prepare in the microwave, and it stays with you all morning.

Always use the large-flake variety (not one-minute or instant oats, as they have already been considerably processed). The body has more to do to metabolize large flake oats, and this slows the digestive process and leaves you feeling fuller longer.

Oatmeal can be endlessly varied by changing the flavour of the fruit yogurt or adding sliced fruit or berries. My wife's favourite oatmeal contains oats, skim milk, unsweetened applesauce, sliced almonds and sweetener. The following is a recipe for my favourite.

OATMEAL (1 SERVING)

½ cup	large-flake oats
1 cup	water or skim milk
½–¾ cup	fat-free fruit yogurt with aspartame
2 tbsp	sliced almonds
	Fresh fruit

Cover oats with water. Microwave on medium setting for 3 minutes. Mix in yogurt, almonds and fresh fruit.

Top the meal off with an orange and a glass of skim milk and you have a delicious breakfast that will stay with you all morning.

HOMEMADE MUESLI (2 SERVINGS)

1 cup	large-flake oats
¾ cup	skim milk
¾ cup	fat-free fruit yogurt with aspartame
2 tbsp	sliced almonds
¾ cup	diced apple or pear, or berries
	Sweetener to taste

In bowl, soak oats in milk. Place in refrigerator overnight. Add yogurt, almonds, fruit and sweetener to taste. Mix well.

COLD CEREAL (1 SERVING)

¾ cup	All-Bran/Bran Buds
¾ cup	skim milk
2 tbsp	sliced almonds
¾ cup	peach or pear slices, or berries
	Sweetener to taste

Mix all ingredients together and enjoy.

A tasty alternative is to add 1/2 cup fruit-flavoured fat-and sugar-free yogurt and cut back a little on the milk.

ON-THE-RUN BREAKFAST (1 SERVING)

Combine:

½ cup	All Bran/Bran Buds
1 cup	fresh fruit
½ cup	cottage cheese (1% or fat-free)
2 tbsp	sliced almonds

And have with:

1 slice	toast, spread with 2 tsp margarine (light) and 1 tbsp double fruit/low sugar spread
1 cup	coffee or tea

OMELETTE (1 SERVING)

2 tsp	olive or canola oil
½ cup	low-cholesterol liquid egg
¼ cup	skim milk

To this basic recipe you can add a variety of fresh vegetables and some cheese flavouring. Crumble and sprinkle a small quantity only of the cheese. Some suggestions are given below. To complete your breakfast include a cup of fresh fruit and a cup of skim milk or 1/2 to 3/4 cup of fat- and sugar-free yogurt.

Italian

To the basic omelette recipe, add:

1 oz	grated skim mozzarella cheese
½ cup	sliced mushrooms
½ cup	tomato purée
	Spices to taste

Mexican

To the basic omelette recipe, add:

½ cup	mixed canned beans
1 cup	chopped red and green peppers
½ cup	sliced mushrooms
	Hot sauce or chili powder to taste

Vegetarian

To the basic omelette recipe, add:

1 oz	grated skim milk cheese
1 cup	broccoli florets
½ cup	sliced mushrooms
½ cup	chopped red and green peppers

Western

To the basic omelette recipe, add:

2 slices	back bacon, lean deli ham or turkey breast, chopped
1	onion, chopped
1 cup	chopped red and green peppers
	Spices to taste

Omelette Preparation

1. Spray olive or canola oil in a non-stick pan over medium heat. Sauté vegetables until tender. Put them on a side plate and keep warm.
2. Mix eggs with milk and pour mixture into pan. Add vegetables (and grated cheese where applicable) as omelette starts to firm.

SCRAMBLED EGGS

Same as omelette recipe, except scramble the egg mixture in the pan.

Lunch

Always have fresh or canned fruit (in water, not syrup), plus a glass of water or (preferably) skim milk with your lunch. Drink decaffeinated coffee or tea with skim milk to suit and no sugar.

Salads

Always ensure you have some protein with your vegetables. Typically, this means adding skinless chicken or turkey, fish, deli-style lean ham, low-fat cottage cheese or beans.

When dining out, always ask for low-fat/light dressings or, if unavailable, oil and vinegar. Always ask for the dressing on the side so you can control the amount. Unfortunately, this means that pre-dressed salads, like Caesar, are out. If you have the time, you can make your own green-light salads at home.

MIXED BEAN SALAD

Use a can of mixed beans—kidney, white, chickpeas and black-eyed peas. (Always rinse before use to remove excess salt.)

Toss with:
> chopped parsley
> diced cucumber
> chopped tomato (optional)
> small amount of pasta shells

Dressing:
>   shallot or red wine vinegar
>   Dijon mustard
>   olive oil
>   pepper

GREEK SALAD

Toss together:
>   iceberg lettuce
>   chopped cucumber
>   chopped tomato
>   olives
>   sliced red onion
>   small amount of crumbled feta (not chunks)

Dressing:
>   dried oregano
>   pepper
>   lemon juice

Eggs

Always ask for an egg substitute or egg whites when dining out. The more vegetables you can incorporate into your egg dish, the better.

Sandwiches

Here are the four G.I. Diet rules for sandwiches:

1. Always ask for whole wheat or whole grain bread. The grittier the bread, the better.

2. Always eat open-faced, discarding the top slice of bread.

3. Try to eat without butter or margarine. Hummus is a great substitute.

4. Avoid regular mayonnaise. Fat-free mayonnaise or yogurt are excellent alternatives.

Wraps

These are growing in popularity and make a good choice in fast-food outlets in particular. Follow the same rules as for sandwiches. Ask for one side of the pita bread to be removed or unwrap and remove it yourself. It still works, but eat carefully.

Soups

The combination of soup and salad is a good one. The soups to go for are the chunky vegetable and barley variety, particularly with beans. Avoid any suggestion of "cream of…"

G.I. Diet Food Guide

BEANS	RED	YELLOW	GREEN
	Baked beans with pork		All beans (canned or dried)
	Broad		Baked beans* (low fat)
			Black-eyed peas
			Chickpeas
			Soybeans
			Split peas

BEVERAGES	RED	YELLOW	GREEN
	Alcoholic drinks**	Diet soft drinks (caffeinated)	Bottled water
	Fruit drinks	Milk (1%)	Club soda
	Milk (whole or 2%)	Most unsweetened juice	Decaffeinated coffee (with skim milk, no sugar)

* Limit quantity.
** In Phase II, a glass of red wine may be had with dinner.

BEVERAGES	RED	YELLOW	GREEN
	Regular coffee	Red wine*	Diet soft drinks (no caffeine)
	Regular soft drinks		Light instant chocolate
	Sweetened juice		Milk (skim)
			Tea (with skim milk, no sugar)

BREADS	RED	YELLOW	GREEN
	Bagels	Pita (whole wheat)	100% stone-ground whole wheat**
	Baguette/ Croissants	Whole grain breads**	Apple Bran Muffins (see p. 89)
	Cake/Cookies		Homemade Granola Bars (see p. 90)
	Corn bread		Whole-grain, high-fibre
	English muffins		breads (2½–3 g fibre
	Hamburger buns		per slice)**
	Hot dog buns		
	Kaiser rolls		
	Melba toast		
	Muffins/Donuts		
	Pancakes/Waffles		
	Pizza		
	Stuffing		
	Tortillas		
	White bread		

* In Phase II, a glass of red wine may be had with dinner.
** Use a single slice only per serving.

CEREALS	RED	YELLOW	GREEN
	All cold cereals except those listed as yellow- or green-light	Shredded Wheat Bran	All-Bran
	Granola		Bran Buds
	Muesli (commercial)		Fibre First
			Homemade Muesli (see p. 74)
			Oat bran
			Porridge (large-flake oatmeal)
			Red River

CEREAL GRAINS	RED	YELLOW	GREEN
	Couscous	Corn	Barley
	Rice (short grain, white, instant)		Buckwheat
			Bulgur
	Rice cakes		Rice (basmati, wild, brown, long grain)

DAIRY	RED	YELLOW	GREEN
	Cheese	Cheese (low fat)	Buttermilk
	Chocolate milk	Cream cheese (light)	Cheese (fat free)
	Cottage cheese (whole or 2%)	Ice cream (low fat)	Cottage cheese (1% or fat free)
	Cream	Milk (1%)	Fruit yogurt (fat and sugar free)
	Cream cheese	Sour cream (light)	Ice cream (low fat and no added sugar, e.g., Breyers Premium Fat
	Ice cream	Yogurt (low fat)	Free, Nestlé's Legend No Added Sugar)
	Milk (whole or 2%)		
	Sour Cream		Milk (skim)
	Yogurt (whole or 2%)		

FATS AND OILS	RED	YELLOW	GREEN
	Butter	Corn oil	Almonds*
	Coconut oil	Mayonnaise (light)	Canola oil*/seed
	Hard margarine	Most nuts	Flax seed
	Lard	Peanut oil	Hazelnuts*
	Mayonnaise	Salad dressings (light)	Macadamia nuts*
	Palm oil	Sesame oil	Mayonnaise (fat free)
	Peanut butter (all varieties)	Soft margarine (non-hydrogenated)	Olive oil*
	Salad dressings (regular)	Sunflower oil	Salad dressings (fat free)
	Tropical oils	Vegetable oils	Soft margarine (non-hydrogenated, light)*
	Vegetable shortening		Vegetable oil sprays

FRUITS	RED	YELLOW	GREEN
FRESH	Cantaloupe	Apricots	Apples
	Honeydew melon	Bananas	Blackberries
	Watermelon	Kiwi	Blueberries
		Mango	Cherries
		Papaya	Grapefruit
		Pineapple	Grapes
			Lemons
			Oranges (all varieties)
			Peaches/Plums
			Pears
			Raspberries
			Strawberries

* Use sparingly.

FRUITS	RED	YELLOW	GREEN
BOTTLED, CANNED, DRIED, FROZEN	All canned fruit in syrup	Canned apricots in juice or water	Applesauce (without sugar)
			Frozen berries
	Applesauce containing sugar	Dried apricots*	Mandarin oranges
			Peaches in juice or water
	Most dried fruit*	Fruit cocktail in juice	Pears in juice or water

JUICES**	RED	YELLOW	GREEN
	Fruit drinks	Apple (unsweetened)	
	Prune	Grapefruit (unsweetened)	
	Sweetened juice	Orange (unsweetened)	
	Watermelon	Pear (unsweetened)	
		Pineapple (unsweetened)	
		Vegetable	

MEAT, POULTRY, FISH, EGGS AND TOFU	RED	YELLOW	GREEN
	Ground beef (more than 10% fat)	Ground beef (lean)	All fish and seafood***
	Hamburgers	Lamb (lean cuts)	Back bacon
	Hot dogs	Pork (lean cuts)	Beef (lean cuts)
	Processed meats	Turkey bacon	Chicken breast (skinless)
	Regular bacon	Whole omega-3 eggs	Ground beef (extra lean)
	Sausages		Lean deli ham

* For baking, it is okay to use a modest amount of dried apricots.

** Whenever possible, eat the fruit rather than drink its juice.

*** Avoid breaded or coated fish and seafood.

MEAT, POULTRY, FISH, EGGS AND TOFU	RED	YELLOW	GREEN
	Whole regular eggs		Low-cholesterol liquid eggs
			Tofu
			Turkey breast (skinless)
			Veal

PASTA*	RED	YELLOW	GREEN
	All canned pastas		Capellini
	Gnocchi		Fettuccine
	Macaroni and cheese		Macaroni
	Noodles (canned or instant)		Penne
	Pasta filled with cheese or meat		Spaghetti/Linguine
			Vermicelli

PASTA SAUCES	RED	YELLOW	GREEN
	Sauces with added meat or cheese	Sauces with vegetables	Light sauces with vegetables
	Sauces with added sugar or sucrose		(no added sugar)

SNACKS	RED	YELLOW	GREEN
	Bagels	Bananas	Almonds**
	Bread	Dark chocolate** (70% cocoa)	Apple Bran Muffins (see p. 89)
	Candy	Ice cream (low-fat)	Applesauce (unsweetened)

* Use whole wheat or protein-enriched pastas if available.

** Limit quantity.

SNACKS	RED	YELLOW	GREEN
	Cookies	Most nuts*	Canned peaches/pears in juice or water
	Crackers	Popcorn (light, microwaveable)	Cottage cheese (1% or fat-free)
	Donuts		Food bars**
	French fries		Fruit yogurt (fat and sugar free)
	Ice cream		Hazelnuts*
	Muffins (commercial)		Homemade Granola Bars (see p. 90)
	Popcorn (regular)		
	Potato chips/		Ice cream (low fat and
	Pretzels		no added sugar, e.g.,
	Raisins		Breyers Premium Fat
	Rice cakes		Free, Nestlé's Legend
	Tortilla chips		No Added Sugar)
	Trail mix		Most fresh fruit
			Most fresh vegetables

SOUPS	RED	YELLOW	GREEN
	All cream-based soups	Chicken noodle	Chunky bean and vegetable soups
	Black bean	Lentil	(e.g., Campbell's
	Green pea	Tomato	Healthy Request,
	Puréed vegetable		Healthy Choice and
	Split pea		Too Good To Be True)

*Limit quantity.
** 180–225 calorie bars, e.g. Power Bars or Balance Bars; ½ bar per serving

SUGAR & SWEETENERS	RED	YELLOW	GREEN
	Corn syrup	Fructose	Aspartame
	Glucose		Equal
	Honey		Splenda
	Molasses		Stevia
	Sugar (all types)		Sugar Twin
			Sweet'N Low

VEGETABLES	RED	YELLOW	GREEN	
	Broad beans	Artichokes	Avocado*	Lettuce (all varieties)
	French fries	Beets	Asparagus	Mushrooms
	Hash browns	Corn	Beans (green/wax)	Olives*
	Parsnips	Potatoes (boiled)	Bell peppers	Onions
	Potatoes (instant)	Pumpkin	Broccoli	Peas
			Brussels sprouts	Peppers (hot)
	Potatoes (mashed or baked)	Squash	Cabbage	Pickles
	Rutabaga	Sweet potatoes	Carrots	Potatoes (boiled new)**
	Turnip	Yams	Cauliflower	Radishes
			Celery	Snow peas
			Cucumbers	Spinach
			Eggplant	Tomatoes
			Leeks	Zucchini

*Limit serving.

** 2-3 served whole or sliced (not mashed) per serving

Dinner

All of the following meal ideas are based on the G.I. Diet portion ratios discussed in chapter 3. Vegetables should take up 50 percent of your plate and should always comprise at least one green vegetable, a mixture of at least two vegetables and a side green salad. Meat, poultry or fish should take up 25 percent of your plate and rice, pasta or potatoes should take up the remaining 25 percent.

I have based the following meal ideas on typical family needs and have modified them along G.I. principles.

Poultry

Basic Preparation

- Apply a vegetable oil spray to a non-stick pan. Sauté 4 oz/120 g whole, sliced or cubed skinless, boneless chicken or turkey breasts per person, until no longer pink. Whole breasts will take a little longer than strips or cubes.

- Set poultry aside.

The cooked breasts can be used in dozens of ways, with various spices and vegetables to enhance the flavour and add variety. Here are just three of the many possibilities:

Asian Stir-fry

1. Stir-fry mixed vegetables, such as carrots, cauliflower, broccoli, mushrooms and snow peas. For convenience, use frozen mixed vegetables.

2. Add salt, pepper, grated ginger root and soy sauce, or prepared sauces such as Too Good To Be True Thai sauce for fast flavour.

3. For colour, add chopped mixed bell peppers (green, yellow and red). Using bags of frozen cut peppers really saves time and effort.

4. Add the chicken or turkey, simmer for 2 minutes and serve.

Italian Chicken

1. Sauté sliced mushrooms, onions and chopped canned Italian tomatoes with a little water to avoid sticking.

2. Season with garlic, oregano and basil (fresh or dried) and simmer vegetables for 5 minutes.

3. Add chicken or turkey, simmer for 2 minutes and serve.

Chicken Curry

1. Sauté sliced onions with 1 tbsp tomato paste and 2 tbsp curry powder (or to taste), for 1 minute.

2. Add 1 cup sliced carrots and 1 cup chopped celery. Sauté 1 minute.

3. Add 1 cup water, 1/2 cup basmati rice, 1 chopped apple and 1/4 cup raisins. Cover and simmer.

4. When liquid is absorbed, add chicken or turkey, heat through and serve.

Fish

Virtually any fish is suitable, but *never* use commercially breaded or battered versions. Salmon and trout are great favourites in our house. Pre-spiced or flavoured varieties are okay, but why pay someone else a whopping premium for what you can easily do yourself?

Basic Preparation

1. Place 4 to 5 oz (120 to 150 g) fish fillets per person in microwaveable dish.

2. Sprinkle fish with 1 to 2 tsp lemon juice and pepper.

3. Cover with plastic wrap, but fold back one corner to allow steam to escape.

4. Microwave for 4 to 5 minutes and serve.

Variations

- Sprinkle fish with fresh or dried herbs such as dill, parsley, basil and tarragon.

- Cook fish on a bed of leeks and onions. Do not use oil.

- Sprinkle fish with a mixture of whole wheat bread crumbs and parsley (1 tbsp per fillet) plus 1 tsp melted light non-hydrogenated margarine.

Serve fish with:

- green beans with almonds or mushrooms

- basmati rice (You can stir some extra vegetables into the rice during the last minute of cooking.) Limit serving size to cover a quarter of the plate—3 tbsp dry (2/3 cup cooked).

- pasta, covering a quarter of the plate—about 35 g dry (3/4 cup cooked)

- an alternative to rice or pasta: boiled new potatoes (2 to 3 per serving) tossed with herbs and a smidgen of olive oil

- mixed vegetables, such as sliced carrots, broccoli or cauliflower florets and halved Brussels sprouts

Meat

Veal and lean deli ham are your best choices. Red meat in general is a yellow-light food, although for pragmatic reasons I've included lean cuts of beef and extra lean ground beef in Phase I. Other red meats such as pork and lamb tend to have a higher fat content. Serving size is critical. Remember, use the palm of your hand or a pack of playing cards as a guide to your portion size. And please do not be alarmed by the apparent modest size of these portions. I had a real problem downsizing my steak at first, but now my stomach reels at the portions served in many restaurants.

Steak

For a complete steak-based meal, try the following:

- Broil or barbecue a fully trimmed lean steak (4 oz/ 120 g per person).

- Sauté sliced onions and mushrooms in a non-stick pan with a little water.

- Microwave, for 3 to 5 minutes, broccoli, asparagus and Brussels sprouts with a little water, seasoned with nutmeg and pepper.

- Boil 3 tbsp dry basmati rice, or 2 to 3 boiled new potatoes per person. Season the potatoes with herbs and a touch of olive oil.

MEAT LOAF

A popular favourite. This version uses extra lean ground beef, which is still relatively high in fat. A lower-fat and better alternative to ground beef is ground turkey or chicken breast.

1 ½ lbs	extra lean ground beef (less than 10 percent fat)
1 cup	tomato juice
½ cup	large-flake oats (uncooked)
1	egg, lightly beaten
½ cup	chopped onion
1 tbsp	Worcestershire sauce
½ tsp	salt (optional)
¼ tsp	pepper

1. Heat oven to 350°F.

2. In a large bowl, combine all ingredients. Mix lightly but thoroughly.

3. Press meat loaf mixture into an 8-x4-inch loaf pan.

4. Bake for 1 hour or until thermometer inserted into centre of meat loaf registers 160°F. (For turkey or chicken, thermometer should register 170°F.)

5. Let stand 5 minutes.

6. Drain any juices before slicing.

CHILI

2 tsp	olive oil
1	large onion, sliced
2	cloves of garlic, minced
½ lb	extra lean ground beef (optional)
2	green peppers, chopped
2 cups	canned tomatoes
3 tbsp	chili powder
½ tsp	cayenne (optional)
½ tsp	salt
¼ tsp	basil
2 cups	water
1 can	red kidney beans, rinsed
1 can	white beans, rinsed

1. Add oil to a deep skillet or saucepan and sauté onion and garlic until nearly tender.
2. Add ground beef, if using, and cook, breaking up with spoon, until browned; drain off any fat.
3. Add green peppers, tomatoes, chili powder, cayenne, salt, basil and water and bring to a boil. Simmer uncovered until it has reached desired consistency (1 to 2 hours).
4. Prior to serving, add the kidney and white beans. You can garnish this chili with chopped tomato, fresh parsley, fresh cilantro and yogurt cheese.*

* You can make yogurt cheese yourself. Drain no-fat yogurt through cheesecloth or a very fine sieve, then refrigerate overnight, covered.

Snacks

Snacks play a critical role between meals by giving you a boost when you most need it. Most popular snack foods are disastrous from a sugar and fat standpoint. Commercial cookies, muffins and candy bars should be avoided at all costs. Fortunately, there are equally satisfying alternatives that are both convenient and low-cost. Never leave home without them.

Below is a list of green-light snacks that require no preparation on your part

- 1 apple, pear, peach or orange
- 4 oz low-fat cottage cheese (1% or less) with 1 tbsp light double fruit preserve
- ¾ cup fat-free fruit yogurt with aspartame
- ½ of a food bar such as a Balance or Power Bar (200 calories; 20–30 g carbohydrates; 12–15 g protein; 5 g fat per bar)

You can also make the following muffins and granola bars and use them as snacks.

APPLE BRAN MUFFINS

¾ cup	All-Bran cereal
1 cup	skim milk
⅔ cup	whole wheat flour
	Sweetener (equivalent to ⅓ cup sugar)
2 tsp	baking powder
½ tsp	baking soda
¼ tsp	salt
1 tsp	allspice
½ tsp	cloves
1 ½ cups	oat bran
⅔ cup	raisins
1	large apple, peeled, cut into ¼-inch cubes
1	egg, lightly beaten
2 tsp	vegetable oil
½ cup	applesauce (unsweetened)

1. Mix the All-Bran and skim milk in a bowl and let stand for a few minutes.

2. In a large bowl, mix the flour, sweetener, baking powder, baking soda, salt and spices. Stir in the oat bran, raisins and apple.

3. In a small bowl, combine the egg, vegetable oil and applesauce. Stir, along with the All-Bran mixture, into the dry ingredients.

4. Spoon the mixture into an oil-sprayed 12-muffin tray. Bake at 350°F for 20 minutes or until lightly browned.

Makes 12 muffins.

HOMEMADE GRANOLA BARS

1 ⅓ cups	whole wheat flour
	Sweetener (equivalent to ⅓ cup sugar)
2 tsp	baking powder
¼ cup	wheat bran
1 tsp	ground cinnamon
1 tsp	allspice
½ tsp	ground ginger
½ tsp	salt (optional)
1 ½ cups	rolled oats
1 cup	apricots (finely chopped)
½ cup	sunflower seeds, shelled
¾ cup	applesauce (unsweetened)
½ cup	apple juice
3	eggs
2 tsp	vegetable oil

1. Line a shallow 8- x 12-inch baking dish with parchment paper.

2. Mix the flour, sweetener, baking powder, bran and spices in a large bowl. Stir in the oats, apricots and sunflower seeds.

3. Mix the applesauce, apple juice, eggs and oil, and add to the flour mixture.

4. Pour into the baking dish and spread evenly.

5. Bake at 400°F for about 15 to 20 minutes, or until lightly browned. Let cool and cut into bars.

Makes 16 bars.

CHAPTER SIX

The Green-Light Glossary

The following is a summary of the most popular green-light foods. For a full green-light list, see colour insert.

Apples	A real staple. Use fresh as a snack or dessert. Unsweetened applesauce is ideal with cereals, or with cottage cheese as a snack.
Barley	An excellent supplement to soups.
Beans (legumes)	If there's one food you can never get enough of, it's beans. These perfect green-light foods are high in protein and fibre and can supplement nearly every meal. Make bean salads or just add beans to any salad. Add to soups, replace some of the meat in casseroles or add to meat loaf. Use as a side vegetable or as an alternative to potatoes, rice or pasta. There's a wide range of canned and frozen beans to check out. Exercise caution with baked beans as the sauce can be high-fat and high-calorie. Check the label for low-fat versions and watch the size of your serving.

Beans have a well-deserved reputation for creating "wind," so be patient until your body adapts—as it will—to your increased consumption.

Bread Most breads are red-light except for 100% stone-ground whole wheat or other whole grain breads with 2 1/2 to 3 grams of fibre per slice. Check labels carefully as the bread industry likes to confuse the unwary. Most bread is made from flour ground by steel rollers, which strip away the bran coating, leaving a very fine powder ideal for producing light, fluffy breads and pastries. Conversely, stone-ground flour is coarser and retains more of its bran coating, so it digests more slowly in your stomach.

Even with 100% stone-ground whole wheat bread, watch your quantity. Use very sparingly in Phase I—no more than one slice per meal.

Cereals Only use large-flake porridge oats, oat bran or high-fibre cold cereals (10 grams of fibre per serving or higher). Though these cereals are not much fun in themselves, you can dress up with fruit (fresh, frozen or canned) or with fruit-flavoured fat- and sugar-free yogurts. This way you can change the menu daily. Use sweetener, not sugar.

Cottage cheese Fat-free or 1% cottage cheese is an excellent low-fat, high-protein food. Add fruit to make a snack or put in salads.

Eggs	By far the best option is whole eggs in liquid form, such as Break Free and Omega Pro, which are both cholesterol- and fat-reduced.
Food bars	Most food or nutrition bars are a dietary disaster, high in carbohydrates and calories but low in protein. These bars are quick sugar fixes on the run. There are a few, such as Balance and Power bars, that have a more equitable distribution of carbohydrates, proteins and fats. Look for 20 to 30 grams of carbohydrates, 10 to 15 grams of protein and 4 to 6 grams of fat. This equals about 220 calories per bar.
	The serving size for a snack is one-half of a bar. Keep one in your office desk or your purse for a convenient on-the-run snack. In an emergency I have been known to have one bar plus an apple and a glass of skim milk for lunch when a proper lunch break was impossible. This is okay in emergencies, but don't make a habit of it.
Grapefruit	One of the top-rated green-light foods. Eat as often as you like.
Hamburgers	These are acceptable but only with extra lean ground beef that has 10% or less fat. Mix in some oat bran to reduce the meat content but keep the bulk. A better option would be to replace the beef with ground turkey or chicken breast. Keep the serving size at 4 ounces; use only half of a whole wheat bun and eat open-faced.

Milk	Use skim only. If you have trouble adjusting, then use 1% and slowly wean yourself off it. The fat you're giving up is saturated (bad) fat. Milk is a terrific snack or meal supplement. I drink two glasses of skim milk a day, at breakfast and lunch.
Nuts	A principal source of "good" fat, which is essential for your health. Almonds are your best choice. Add them to cereals, salads and desserts.
Oat bran	An excellent high-fibre additive to baking as a partial replacement for flour, or as a hot cereal.
Oatmeal	If you haven't had oatmeal since you were a kid, now's the time to revisit it. Large-flake, or old-fashioned, oatmeal is the breakfast of choice, with the added advantage for your heart of lowering cholesterol. A somewhat cynical colleague recently decided to take my advice about the G.I. Diet, but only a meal at a time, starting with oatmeal for breakfast. His oatmeal-based green-light breakfast has so far netted him ten pounds of weight loss! He's since thrown caution to the wind and is now a convert to three green-light meals a day. Personally, I often have an oatmeal porridge snack with unsweetened applesauce and sweetener on the weekends.
Oranges	Whole or in segments, fresh oranges are excellent as snacks, on cereal and especially at breakfast. A glass of orange juice has 2 1/2 times as many calories as a whole orange, so avoid the juice and stick with the real thing.

Pasta	Whole wheat pastas are preferable. But there are always two golden rules. First, do not overcook; *al dente* (some firmness to the bite) is important. Second, serving size: pasta is a side dish and should never occupy more than a quarter of your plate. It *must not* form the basis of the meal, as it most commonly does nowadays in North America, with disastrous results for waistlines and hips.
Peaches/pears	Terrific snacks, desserts or additions to breakfast cereal. Use fresh, or canned in juice or water.
Potatoes	The only form of potatoes that is acceptable even on an occasional basis is boiled new potatoes. New potatoes have a low starch content, unlike larger, more mature potatoes that have been allowed to build their starch levels. All other forms of potato—baked, mashed or fried—are strictly red light. Limit quantity to two or three per serving.
Rice	There is a wide range in the G.I. ratings for various types of rice, most of which are red light. The best rice is basmati or long grain, and brown is better than white. If rice is sticky, with the grains clumping together, don't use it. Similarly, don't overcook rice; the more it's cooked, the more glutinous and therefore unacceptable it becomes. The rule, then, is eat only slightly undercooked basmati rice, which is readily available at your supermarket.

Sweeteners	There has been a tremendous amount of misinformation circulating about artificial sweeteners—all of which has proven groundless. The sugar industry rightly saw these new products as a threat and has done its best to bad-mouth them. Use sweeteners to replace sugar wherever possible. For a medical overview, read about sugar substitutes on the U.S. Food and Drug Administration's Web site, **www.fda.gov**.
Yogurt	Non-fat, fruit-flavoured yogurt sweetened with aspartame is a near perfect green-light product. It's an ideal snack food on its own, or a flavourful addition to breakfast cereal—especially porridge oats—and to fruit for dessert. Our fridge is always full of it, in half a dozen delicious flavours. In fact, my shopping cart is so full of yogurt containers that fellow shoppers frequently stop me to ask if they are on special!
Yogurt Cheese	A wonderful substitute for cream in desserts or in main dishes like chili (see recipe on page 87).

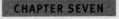

CHAPTER SEVEN

Phase II

Congratulations! You've achieved your new weight target!

Now is the moment to go back to page 30 and complete the chart you started a few months ago. Compare what you ate then with your current diet. I promise you'll be amazed at the change.

This may be hard to believe, but when I had reached my target weight—I lost twenty-two pounds, and three inches off my waist—I had to make a conscious effort to eat more in order to avoid losing more weight. My wife said I was entering the "gaunt zone"!

Phase II Meals and Snacks

The objective in Phase II is to increase the number of calories you consume so that you maintain your new weight. Remember the equation: food energy ingested must equal energy expended to keep weight stable. For the past few weeks you've been taking in less food energy than you've been expending, using your fat reserves to make up the shortfall. Now we make up that deficit by taking in some extra food energy or calories.

Two words of caution. First, your body has become accustomed to doing with fewer calories and has to a certain extent adapted. The result is that your body is more efficient than it was in the bad old days when it had more food energy than it could use. Second, your new lower weight requires fewer calories to function. For example, if you lost 10 percent of your weight, then you need 10 percent fewer calories for your body to function.

Combining a more efficient body, which requires less energy to operate, with a lower weight, which requires fewer calories, means that you need only a marginal increase in food energy to balance the energy in/energy out equation. The biggest mistake most people make when coming off a diet is assuming that they can now consume a much higher calorie level than their new bodies really need. The bottom line is that Phase II is only marginally different than Phase I. Phase II provides you with an opportunity to make small adjustments to portions and add new foods from the yellow-light category. All the fundamentals of the Phase I plan, however, remain inviolable. The following are some suggestions for how you might wish to modify your new eating pattern in Phase II.

Breakfast

- Increase cereal serving size, e.g., from 1/2 to 2/3 cup oatmeal.

- Add a slice of 100% whole grain toast and a pat of margarine.

- Double up on the sliced almonds on cereals.

- Help yourself to an extra slice of back bacon.

- Have a glass of juice now and then.

- Add one of the forbidden fruits—a banana or raisins—to your cereal.

Lunch

I suggest you continue to eat lunch as you did in Phase I. This is the one meal that contained some compromises in the weight-loss portion of the program since it is a meal most of us buy each day.

Dinner

- Add another boiled new potato (from two or three to three or four).

- Increase the rice or pasta serving from 3/4 to 1 cup.

- Have a 6-ounce steak instead of your regular 4-ounce. Make this a special treat, not a habit.

- Eat a few more olives and nuts, but watch the serving size as these are calorie heavyweights.

- Try a cob of sweet corn with a dab of non-hydrogenated margarine.

- Add a slice of whole grain rye or pumpernickel bread.

- Have a lean cut of lamb or pork (maximum 4-ounce serving).

Snacks

WARNING: Strictly watch quantity or serving size.

- light microwave popcorn (maximum 2 cups)

- nuts, maximum eight to ten

- a square or two of bittersweet chocolate (see next page)

- a banana

- one scoop of low-fat ice cream

Chocolate

To many of us, the idea of a chocolate-free world is abhorrent. The good news is that some chocolate, in limited quantities, is acceptable.

Most chocolate contains large quantities of saturated fat and sugar, making it quite fattening. However, chocolate with a high cocoa content (70%) has less fat and less sugar. So, a square or two of rich, dark, bittersweet chocolate, nibbled slowly or better yet, dissolved in the mouth gives us chocoholics the fix we need. This high-cocoa chocolate is available at specialty stores and can even be found in some supermarkets.

Alcohol

Now is the moment you've been waiting for. In Phase II a daily glass of wine, preferably red and with dinner, is not only allowed—it's encouraged! Recently, there has been a flood of research into the benefits of alcohol on heart disease. It has been found that red wine, rich in flavonoids, when drunk in moderation (a glass a day) has a demonstrable benefit in reducing the risk of heart attack and stroke. The theory that says if one glass is good for you, two must be better is tempting but not true. One glass gives the optimum benefit.

As with coffee, if you're only going to have a glass of wine a day, make it a great one. My eldest son, who is a computer programmer in Seattle and lives a lifestyle I can only dream about, took me at my word on wine and gave me a subscription to the *Wine Spectator*. It's proven to be the most costly present I've ever received, as a whole new world of wine and wine ratings has opened up to me. My $10-a-bottle ceiling for special occasions has now doubled or tripled, though it's all being rationalized: I'm drinking less, so I can afford the extravagance!

As a beer aficionado, I like to drink the occasional beer as an alternative to wine. This habit has recently received an endorsement from a group of scientists, who reported in late 1999 that beer (in moderation) would reduce cholesterol and thus heart disease; delay menopause; and reduce the risk of several cancers. They also noted that beer has anti-inflammatory and anti-allergic properties, plus a positive effect on bone density. Personally, I worry about any product being touted as the wonder cure for all our ills, but clearly a glass of beer with supper is likely to do more good than harm.

If you do drink alcohol, always have it with your meal. Food slows down the absorption of alcohol, thereby minimizing its impact.

The Way You Will Eat for the Rest of Your Life

With all these new options in Phase II, the temptation may be to overdo it. If the pounds start to reappear, simply revert to the Phase I plan for a while and you'll be astonished at how quickly your equilibrium is restored.

Phase II is the way you will eat for the rest of your life. You will look and feel better, have more energy and experience none of those hypoglycemic lows. One reason, of course, that you have more energy is that you're not carrying around all that surplus fat. It might be fun to resurrect the backpack and load it up with the weight you've just lost. Carry it around on your back for an hour or two and then rejoice that you don't have to carry it around for the rest of your life! Whenever your resolve wavers, reach for the backpack. It's a marvellous motivator.

The opportunity to succeed is in your hands. I've tried to give you a simple yet motivating plan that will not leave you hungry, tired or confused. It's all here in the book; the rest is up to you.

So, put on the backpack for a couple of hours, clear out the pantry and drive to the supermarket. Remember to park as far as possible from the entrance and enjoy the extra walk. Everything starts with a first step!

CHAPTER EIGHT

Exercise

Conventional wisdom has it that exercise is an essential component of a weight loss program. Recent research findings strongly indicate that this is, in fact, *not* the case. Though any increase in an individual's level of activity is bound to burn up more calories, the net impact over the relatively short weight-loss period (typically twelve to twenty-four weeks) is small. However, over the long haul, to maintain your new weight, exercise is an important contributor. For example, if you were to walk briskly for half an hour a day, seven days per week, you would burn up calories equalling twenty pounds of fat per year. This means that in Phase I, exercise is not essential to your weight-loss program, but it is an important consideration in Phase II, where you maintain your new weight.

Exercise has been an important part of my life since the age of thirty-eight, when I was humbled by my seven-year-old son. He challenged me to a run around the block—and he won soundly. I recognize that exercise is a subject many people don't want to hear about. Nevertheless, before you skip it totally, read the box below. If you still aren't convinced you should read on, then this chapter is not for you.

REGULAR EXERCISE WILL:
1. assist in weight maintenance;
2. dramatically reduce your risk of heart disease, stroke, diabetes and osteoporosis;
3. improve your mental well-being and boost your self-esteem;
4. help you to sleep better.

For those couch potatoes who have been driven by curiosity to read this far, stay with us and see if the following objections to regular exercise sound like your own: "It's painful," "It's boring," "I don't have the time." We are going to address all three complaints head-on.

Firstly, let's look at the pain or discomfort excuse. This probably comes from an experience where you've tried to do too much too soon. The world's basements are full of exercise equipment purchased in a moment of excessive enthusiasm—probably coupled with some New Year's resolutions. A few weeks later, aching muscles, a sore bottom and burning lungs have relegated that exercise bike or other exotic machine to the deep, dark storeroom where we put things that "may be useful later." Sound familiar?

To avoid pain, you must start small and work yourself up. Ten years ago I was an active jogger, running twenty-five to thirty miles a week. Unfortunately, I developed a back disc problem (totally unrelated to jogging) and it was nine years before I ventured out again. Though I kept reasonably trim during that nine-year period, I couldn't believe the problems that my re-entry to jogging created. Day One saw me enthusiastically bounding out the door in my beautiful new running shoes. Half a mile later I stopped in a wheezing heap, lungs burning, knees aching, calf muscles in spasm. You're probably thinking "serves him right," confirming for yourself that exercise is a painful option.

The reason I'm relating this story is that I had to learn the hard way. Jogging is a wonderful exercise, but it places a high demand on your body, particularly if you're over forty. Since I fell into that age category, I had to find an alternative exercise that required less physical effort and was more in tune with the realities of my aging body. I decided to start walking. Nearly everyone can walk, and if you start small and work yourself up, it is pain free (see page 112).

The second objection to exercise is boredom. I am very sympathetic to this one. While some exercises like jogging, walking and bicycling are, by their outdoor nature, rarely boring—unless people, and what they do and where they live, are of no interest to you—Canadian winters can be a disincentive. The nine years I spent working out on my exercise bike and ski machine in the basement were more of a challenge. Granted, this wasn't my only option. Many people use fitness clubs for both the motivation

("I've paid my fee, so I'd better use it") as well as the social interaction and mutual encouragement. One or two of the well-heeled have personal trainers, but this is an unrealistic option for most of us.

Instead, I chose the basement, as there was no fitness facility nearby. My solution to the inherent boredom came via an ancient TV abandoned by the children as they left the nest, and an early "replay only" VCR. I recorded those shows and films that ran between midnight and six a.m. on the family VCR, and they provided my entertainment. I pedalled and skied my way through James Bond movies, build-your-own-cottage shows and Jacques Cousteau undersea documentaries. There was never a boring moment. In fact I sometimes became so engrossed in the shows that I exercised far beyond my scheduled time allocation. Indoors, a little ingenuity (which could be as simple as putting on a Walkman), can help make workouts more interesting.

The last objection is lack of time. There are 336 thirty-minute blocks of time each week. Take 2 percent, or seven, of these blocks and use one each day. This can hardly be an unreasonable allocation of your time, especially when you consider the benefits: a slimmer, fitter, healthier you! Thirty minutes a day should be your target, though I know that many of you will want to increase this allocation once you feel the remarkable improvements that such a modest time commitment can bring.

As far as what time of day you should exercise is concerned, there are two clear camps: those who are at their best first thing in the morning and those who warm up during the day to hit their peak in the evening. I strongly suggest you align your exercise activity with whichever camp you fall into. In our household I'm the morning person, who cannot imagine exercising at the end of the day as my watchspring winds down. My wife, conversely, dreads the mornings but is a going concern by the time we get home in the evening. Needless to say, we don't exercise together. So choose your best time—either bounding out of bed to greet the dawn or exercising away accumulated tensions at the end of the day. Either way, exercise will be an enjoyable component of your daily routine.

Many people find that as their level of fitness increases, they sleep better and wake up feeling more refreshed, taking less time to drag themselves from bed. This in itself frees up more time for exercise, resulting in even less of a draw upon your day.

When referring to "exercise," we're talking about aerobic, or cardio, exercise, which boosts the heart rate and causes you to breathe harder. But before we look at exercise options and getting started, let's talk further about why we're doing this.

Weight Loss and Maintenance

One thing we need to get straight right off: exercise is *not* a substitute for dieting. Dieting will have a far greater impact on weight loss than exercise. What brought home this point to me was the annual rowing race between Oxford and Cambridge Universities on the river Thames. Rowing, along with water polo, is rated as the toughest physical endurance test for the body, and the race is over four miles long. It amazed me to find out that each rower burns the calorie equivalent of only one bar of chocolate during the race! Obviously an enormous expenditure of energy is needed to offset our poor dietary habits. But exercise is an essential complement to diet. Together, the two will give you optimum weight loss and, even more importantly, maintain your new healthy weight.

Exercise works in exactly the same way as diet to reduce or control weight. The more energy (calories) you expend than you take in, the more your body will use up your energy reserve (fat) to make up the shortfall. Exercise burns calories. In fact, every action you perform uses calories. So, climbing the stairs instead of taking the elevator to your office, getting off the bus a stop or two early, or parking as far away as possible from the mall or supermarket entrance will require extra activity over your normal routine and thereby consume extra calories. As we noted earlier, if you were to walk briskly for half an hour a day, you would lose twenty pounds a year automatically. How come? Well, a brisk half-hour walk consumes approximately 200 extra calories. Multiply that by 365 days and you get 72,000 calories, or 20 pounds (1 pound = 3,600 calories).

Note: the thirty-minute (2.5-km) walk that burns 200 calories is based on a 150-pound person. Heavier people will burn more calories in thirty minutes, and lighter people will burn fewer. A 200-pound person will burn 220 calories, a 130-pound person 175 calories. And the more briskly you walk, the more calories you will consume.

Exercise has two further benefits on weight loss and control. First, exercise increases your metabolism—the rate at which you burn up calories—*even after you've finished exercising*. In other words, the benefits stay with you all day. Exercise in the morning is particularly beneficial as it sets the pace for your metabolism for the day.

A second bonus is that exercise builds muscle mass. Starting at the age of twenty-five, the body loses 1.5 percent of its muscle mass each year. High-protein diets can accelerate that loss. By exercising muscles on a regular basis, the loss can be minimized or reversed. And why is that important? Because the larger your muscles, the more energy (calories) they use. When you're at rest, or even asleep in bed, your muscles are using energy. So keeping or building muscle mass really helps you to burn calories and lose weight.

Though regular exercise will help minimize muscle loss, it is resistance exercises that actually build muscle mass. Resistance exercises are those where weights, elastic bands or hydraulics are used for muscles to pull or push against. Most of you are probably cringing at the thought of sweating body builders doing endless painful workouts with massive barbells and other daunting equipment. As we will show a little later, though, it does not have to be like that. A few simple exercises will do wonders to tone and restore those flabby muscles.

We will deal with the other health benefits of exercise in chapter 9 when we look at the impact of weight on your health, in particular on heart disease and stroke, which accounts in North America for four deaths out of every ten.

Getting Started

Now that you're convinced exercise is for you, how do you go about getting started?

1. Select an exercise that suits you. The fastest way to abandon an exercise program is to do something you don't enjoy. It is best to select an exercise that uses the largest muscle groups, that is, the legs, abdominals and lower back. These burn more calories because of their sheer size. Walking, jogging and biking are excellent choices.

2. Get support from family and friends. If possible, find a like-minded buddy so you have support.

3. Set goals and keep a record. A clippable exercise log (see page 157) is included to help keep you on track. Put it on the fridge or in the bathroom.

4. Check with your doctor to ensure that he/she supports your plan.

Now let's review your options.

Outdoor Activities

Walking

This is by far the simplest and, for most people, the easiest exercise program to start and maintain. Thirty minutes a day, seven days a week, should be your target. If you add an hour-long walk on the weekend, you can take a day off during the week. As mentioned before, we're talking about brisk walking—not speed walking or ambling. It must increase your heart and breathing rate, but never exercise to the point where you cannot find the breath to converse with a partner.

You don't need any special clothing or equipment except a pair of comfortable cushioned shoes or sneakers. And walking is rarely boring since you can keep changing routes and watch the world go by as you exercise. Walk with a friend for company and mutual support, or go solo and commune with nature and your own thoughts. I do my best thinking of the day on my morning walk. This is not surprising when you realize how much extra oxygen-fresh blood is pumping through your brain.

A great idea is to incorporate your walking into your daily commute to work. I get off the bus three stops early on my way to and from work. Those three stops are equal to about 2.5 kilometres, so I'm walking about 5 kilometres per day! If you drive to work, try parking your car about 2.5 kilometres away and walk to your job. You may even find cheaper parking farther out.

Jogging

This exercise is similar to walking, but more care is needed with footwear to protect joints from damage. The advantage of jogging over walking is that it approximately doubles the number of calories burned in the same period of time—400 calories for jogging versus 200 for brisk walking over a thirty-minute period. While walking, try jogging for a few yards and see if this is for you. It will get your heart rate up, which is great for heart health. The heart is basically a muscle, and like all muscles it thrives on being exercised—in general, the more the better. If jogging is for you, then this could arguably be the simplest and most effective method of exercise, as it uses personal time efficiently, can be done any time, anywhere, and is inexpensive.

Hiking

Another version of walking is cross-country hiking. Because this usually involves varying terrain, especially hills and valleys, you use up more calories—about 50 percent more than for brisk walking. The reason is that, going uphill, you use considerably more energy as your body literally has to lift its own weight from the bottom to the top. You try hauling 150 to 200 pounds up a hill and you'll get some idea of the extra effort your body has to make. Hiking is a great deal of fun, too, especially on weekends when you can get out of town. It also provides a change of pace from your regular walking or jogging routine.

Bicycling

Like walking, jogging and hiking, bicycling is a fun way to burn up those calories, and it is almost as effective as jogging. Again, other than the cost of the bike, it's inexpensive and can be done almost anywhere and any time. It can also be done indoors during winter months with a stationary bike.

Bicycling offers another good change of pace from your regular routine. I find it gives me a chance to visit all sorts of communities outside my normal walking range.

Other Outdoor Activities

Rollerblading, ice skating, skiing (especially cross-country), snowshoeing and swimming (in a lake or pool) are good alternatives to or changes of pace from any of the above activities. They are similar to biking in terms of energy consumption.

Sports

Though most sports are terrific calorie burners, they usually cannot be part of a regular routine. Most require other people, equipment and facilities, all of which mitigate against a continuing, regular exercise program. But again, they can be an excellent top-up or boost to your regular program. Popular sports such as golf (no golf cart, please), tennis, basketball and softball are excellent adjuncts to a basic exercise program. But they are not a substitute for a five-to-seven-days-a-week regular schedule.

Indoor Activities

Many of you will be muttering by now about how this would all sound fine if we lived in California, but get real, this is Canada; you can't do many of these activities for half the year. Though this is true in general, if you are properly attired the walking/jogging season can be extended to cover most of the year except for those days when no one wants to go outside.

The alternative is either a home gym or a fitness club. The latter is an easy option these days in most larger communities. Clubs offer not only a wide range of sophisticated equipment, but also mutual support from friends and expert advice from staff.

If a fitness club isn't convenient or those Lycra-clad young things make you uncomfortable, the simple alternative is to exercise at home. The best and least expensive equipment is a stationary exercise bike. The latest models work on magnetic resistance rather than the old friction strap around the flywheel. This gives a smoother action with better tension adjustment. Most important, they are quiet, which is crucial if you want to be able to listen to music or watch TV. (The alternative is to turn up the volume until the neighbours complain, or use a headset.)

You can easily pay into the thousands for a bike with all the fancy trimmings, one that is designed for use in a fitness club, but in reality the $250 to $350 machine will work fine. Just be sure it has smooth, adjustable tension and proper seat height, then plug in that late-night movie or your favourite soap and get pedalling. You'll be amazed how quickly the minutes fly by. I've frequently gone way over my scheduled time as I've become immersed in the screen action! Twenty minutes on the bike will give you the same calorie consumption as thirty minutes of brisk walking.

If biking is not for you, try a treadmill. These can be expensive, and beware the lower-end models that cannot take the pounding. Expect to pay about $700 to $1,000, and ensure that the incline of the track can be raised and lowered for a better workout.

Both bikes and treadmills can simulate outdoor walking, jogging, hiking or biking in the comfort of your own home. I use both of these machines but have added a cross-country ski machine, which has the advantage of working the upper body as well. Ski machines are generally less expensive than treadmills but cost more than stationary bikes. They also burn a considerably higher number of

---

Note: Most authorities support the notion that any extra activity is better than none at all. We have no argument with that, but experience shows that if people start substituting washing the car or throwing the ball for the dog as alternatives to a regular brisk exercise program, then the program does not work. By all means garden, wash the windows or whatever else you like, but please do not fool yourself into thinking that this will have a significant impact on your weight loss or maintenance program.

calories (similar to jogging) because they use arms and shoulders as well as legs—almost the perfect all-body workout machine.

There are several other more specialized options, such as stair step or rowing machines, but they are not for everyone. They are also quite expensive, so make sure you try them out first at a fitness club or with a co-operative retailer.

Resistance Training

It's now time to pay some attention to rebuilding your muscle mass. Remember that after age forty, you will lose between four and six pounds of muscle every decade. That's four to six pounds of calorie-consuming muscle. Muscles burn up energy even when idle. Let me illustrate this point. As a student I pumped gas during one of my vacations. One day a pre-war Bentley drove in and the owner asked me to fill her right to the top. He left the car running and went to the washroom. The car was filled through a large pipe that stuck about eighteen inches out of the gas tank. I was not able to fill the tank to the top of the pipe because the level kept dropping with every beat of the huge twelve-cylinder engine. I finally had to ask the owner to switch off the engine so I could finally top it up! The lesson is that, like the Bentley, bigger muscles consume more energy than smaller muscles, even when idling.

Resistance training equipment can range from the complex and expensive to the simple and inexpensive. Home gyms are a popular option for a few hundred dollars and up. For most people, however, there are much simpler methods—free weights or (my own preference) rubber bands. Dynaband and Thera-Band are two popular choices. The latter I find particularly useful as it comes in varying thicknesses, offering increasing levels of resistance as you regain and build your muscle strength.

Thera-Band comes in rolls of six-inch-wide rubber strips, in different colours for different thicknesses (the thicker the band, the more resistance to stretching). The big advantage of this form of resistance training is that it's inexpensive ($10 to $20), so lightweight that you can take it anywhere, and progressive, providing a psychological boost as you trade up to the next level of resistance (there are eight levels). You'll find a list of suggested exercises in Appendix V.

After two years of use I've now reached the maximum resistance level with Thera-Band, so I've added some five-pound wrist and ankle weights to the workout. These resistance rubber bands and weights are available at surgical supply stores and many exercise equipment retailers.

Try a few resistance exercises, concentrating on the larger muscle groups—your legs, arms and upper chest. These are the muscles that will give you the biggest bang by burning up the most calories. The resistance exercises should add to your other regular exercise regimen, not replace it. Muscle-building exercise is strictly complementary to regular get-your-body-moving exercise. Using both types of exercise together will work far better than either one alone. And resistance exercises are best done every other day, leaving time for your muscles to recuperate.

For a complete exercise overview, including instructions for warm-up, strengthening and stretching exercises, see Appendix V.

TO SUM UP:

1. A regular exercise program will accelerate weight loss and help you maintain a desired weight. It will also improve your health (especially heart health), make you feel good and allow you to sleep better. It will be the best thirty-minute-a-day investment you'll ever make.

2. Choose an activity that suits your personality and your schedule.

3. Stick to it. Make it part of your life at least five days a week—preferably every day.

CHAPTER NINE

Health

Foods are, in effect, drugs. They have a powerful influence on our health, well-being and emotional state. We take in food four or five times a day, usually with more thought for taste than for nutritional value. It would be incomprehensible to take drugs on the same basis.

The right foods can help you maintain your health, extend your lifespan, give you more energy, and make you feel good and sleep better. Couple that with exercise and you are doing all you can to keep healthy, fit and alert. The rest is a matter of genes and luck.

We'll now examine the role of diet and exercise in preventing diseases.

Heart Disease and Stroke

Given that I was the president of the Heart and Stroke Foundation of Ontario for fifteen years, it is hardly surprising that I'm starting with these diseases. However, there is a more important reason: heart disease and stroke cause 40 percent of North American deaths. Remarkably, this is evidence of progress. When I first joined the Foundation, the figure was close to 50 percent.

This is a good news, bad news story. The good news is that advances in surgery, drug therapies and emergency services have saved many lives. The bad news is that twice as many deaths could have been averted if only we had reduced our weight, exercised regularly and quit smoking. Though the smoking rate for adults has dropped sharply (unfortunately, we cannot say the same for teens), we are eating more and exercising less, leading inevitably to a more obese and unhealthy population. It's been calculated that if we led even a moderate lifestyle, we could halve the carnage from these diseases. Though heart disease, like most cancers, is primarily a disease of old age, nearly half of those who suffer heart attacks are under the age of sixty-five.

A familiar refrain that I have heard many times is, "Why worry? If I have a heart attack, today's medicine will save me." It might well save you from immediate death, but what most people do not realize is that the heart is permanently damaged after an attack. The heart cannot repair itself because its cells do not reproduce. (Ever wonder why you cannot get cancer of the heart? That's the reason.) After the damage sustained during a heart attack, the heart has to work harder to compensate—but it never can. It slowly degenerates under this stress, and patients finally "drown" as blood circulation fails and the lungs fill with liquid. Congestive heart failure is a dreadful way to die, so make sure you do everything you can to avoid having a heart attack in the first place.

With regard to diet, the simple fact is that the fatter you are, the more likely it is you will suffer a heart attack or stroke. The two key factors that link heart disease and stroke to diet are cholesterol and hypertension (high blood pressure). I promised at the beginning of this book that I was not going to dwell on the complexities of the science of nutrition; it's the outcome of this science that's important. However, a little science is helpful to understand the role and importance of both hypertension and cholesterol.

Hypertension, or high blood pressure, is the harbinger of both heart disease and stroke. High blood pressure puts more stress on the arterial system and causes it to age and deteriorate more rapidly, ultimately leading to arterial damage, blood clots, and heart attack or stroke. Excess weight has a major bearing on high blood pressure. A Canadian study in 1997 found that obese adults, aged eighteen to fifty-five, had a five to thirteen times greater risk of hypertension. A further study demonstrated that a lower fat diet coupled with a major increase in fruits and vegetables (eight to ten servings a day) lowered blood pressure. The moral: lose weight and eat more fruits and vegetables to help reduce your blood pressure levels. In other words, adopt the G.I. Diet.

Cholesterol is essential to your body's metabolism. However, high cholesterol is a problem as it's the key ingredient in the plaque that can build up in your arteries, eventually cutting off the blood supply to your heart (causing heart attack) or your brain (leading to stroke). To make things more complicated, there are two forms of cholesterol: HDL (good) cholesterol and LDL (bad) cholesterol. The idea is to boost the HDL level while depressing the LDL level. (Remember it this way: HDL is **H**eart's **D**elight **L**evel and LDL is **L**eads to **D**eath **L**evel.)

The villain in raising LDL levels is saturated fat, which is usually solid at room temperature and is found primarily in meat and whole milk and food products. Conversely, polyunsaturated and monounsaturated fats not only lower LDL levels but actually boost HDL. The moral: make sure some fat is included in your diet, but make sure it's the right fat. (Refer to chapter 1 for the complete rundown on fat.)

Diabetes

Diabetes is the kissing cousin of heart disease in that more people die from heart complications arising from diabetes than from diabetes alone. And diabetes rates are skyrocketing: they are expected to double in the next ten years.

The principal causes of the most common form of diabetes, Type 2, are obesity and lack of exercise, and the current epidemic is strongly correlated to the obesity trend. The most dramatic illustration of this link appears in Canada's Native population, where in some communities diabetes affects nearly half the adult population.

Before the Europeans colonized North America, the Native peoples lived in a state of feast or famine. When there was an abundance of food, plant or animal, it was stored in the body as fat. In lean times, such as winter, the body depleted these fat supplies. As a result their bodies developed a "thrift gene," with those who stored and utilized their food most effectively being the survivors— a classic Darwinian exercise in survival of the fittest. When you take away the need to hunt or to harvest food—that is, the need to exercise—and replace it with a trip to the supermarket whenever food is required, the result is inevitable: a massive increase in obesity and, with it, diabetes.

Foods with a low G.I., which release sugar more slowly into the bloodstream, appear to play a major role in helping diabetics control their disease. Thus the G.I. Diet provides an opportunity both to lose weight and to assist in the management of the disease. Prevention, however, is far preferable, so get right into your G.I. Diet program and get those pounds off.

Cancer

The connection between diet and cancer is less distinct. However, a recent global report by the American Institute for Cancer Research concluded that 30 to 40 percent of cancers are directly linked to dietary choices. Its key recommendation is that individuals should choose a predominantly plant-based diet that includes a variety of vegetables, fruit and grains—the G.I. Diet in a nutshell.

CHAPTER TEN

Supplements

As a young advertising account executive in the United Kingdom, I was briefed by a nutritionist on vitamin supplements, which Miles Labs was planning to introduce into England. The nutritionist was skeptical about the readiness of the British for these American-style multivitamin therapies and whether in fact we even needed them. Her comment—"our sewers contain the richest concentration of vitamins in the country"—still resounds in my head whenever the question of vitamins and other food supplements comes up.

There is a great deal of truth in what she said. Most of us get at least the minimum recommended levels of most vitamins and minerals from our diet. There is increasing evidence, however, that the usual RDA (Recommended Daily Allowance) may be insufficient in certain specific instances. This is a dynamic area of nutrition research and very susceptible to change as new data pours in on a daily basis. Based on our present knowledge, here are some guidelines that may be helpful.

Vitamin B

There is growing evidence that vitamin B, or more specifically B6, B12 and folic acid, are key ingredients in combatting a chemical called homocysteine, which attacks your arteries. This substance is triggered by digesting animal protein, which again suggests that high-protein diets can be dangerous to your health.

Because excessive doses of some B vitamins can be dangerous, the levels in most one-a-day multivitamins (20 mcg B12, 2 mg B6, 400 mcg folic acid) are quite sufficient as a top-up to any possible deficiencies in your diet.

Vitamin C

This is certainly the most popular vitamin sold, mainly because of its association with cold prevention and reduction. Though there is little evidence to support that traditional claim, we do know that vitamin C is critical to muscles, ligaments and joints.

While the G.I. Diet, with its emphasis on fresh fruit and vegetables, will certainly cover your basic vitamin C requirements, a top-up through a one-a-day multivitamin may help.

Vitamin D

This is the true sunshine vitamin, and not vitamin C as the Florida ads suggest. Though vitamin D is prevalent in milk and fatty fish, our body can only produce vitamin D itself when exposed to sunshine. For Canadians sunshine is a scarce commodity in winter, and since we should be lathered in sunscreen during our brief summer we are unable to capitalize on this vitamin self-generation.

Vitamin D is important because it facilitates the processing of calcium for your bones. This is critical for people over fifty, especially women, in order to prevent osteoporosis. A shortage of vitamin D can also bring on aches and pains similar to symptoms of arthritis.

Again, the G.I. Diet, with its emphasis on low-fat milk and fish, will help, but it won't hurt to top up with a multivitamin, which normally contains the recommended daily level of 400 IU.

Vitamin E

This became the wonder vitamin of the 1990s when it was suggested that it could reduce heart disease, Alzheimer's and certain cancers. There are many significant population studies currently underway, though recent heart disease reports have been somewhat contradictory.

Vitamin E is the one principal vitamin that is underrepresented in most multivitamins. The recommended daily dosage is 100 to 400 IU, whereas most multivitamins contain only 30 to 50 IU. The G.I. Diet will give you a good natural supply of vitamin E, which is found in vegetable oils and nuts (both also sources of "good" fat). However, you would require a significant intake of these vegetable fats to realize the recommended levels. Taking a 400 IU vitamin E supplement is therefore a good idea and carries little risk. Many cardiologists take this supplement, which is as good a recommendation as any.

Fish Oil

There is one oil in particular that has been found to have significant positive health benefits, particularly for your heart. The oil is called omega-3, and it is a fatty acid found primarily in coldwater fish, salmon in particular, as well as in canola and flax seed. As most of us are unlikely to consume salmon on a daily basis, salmon oil is available in capsule form in any pharmacy. I take a couple at breakfast (2000 mg) every day. The research evidence supporting omega-3 is overwhelming and much of it is Canadian, stemming from studies of the Inuit, who do not eat what we consider a heart-healthy diet, with loads of animal fat and virtually no fruit or vegetables. However, the coldwater fish they consume, rich in omega-3, appears to give them protection against heart disease.

TO SUM UP:
The G.I. Diet almost certainly contains sufficient vitamins to meet your daily needs. However, if you are at all concerned, a one-a-day multivitamin offers cheap and risk-free insurance. An extra vitamin E pill is optional, but keep your ears and eyes open to new research on this front. If heart health is a particular concern, omega-3 oil capsules are a good idea.

Appendix I

Green-Light Pantry Guide

PANTRY	FRIDGE	FREEZER
BAKING/COOKING	**DAIRY**	**DAIRY**
Whole wheat flour	Milk (skim)	Ice cream (fat free and no added sugar)
Baking powder/soda	Fruit yogurt (fat and sugar free)	
Cocoa	Buttermilk	
Wheat bran	Cottage cheese (1%)	
Sliced almonds		
Dried apricots		
BEANS (CANNED)	**FRUIT**	**MEAT/POULTRY/FISH**
Baked (low fat)	Apples	(see Fridge)
Mixed salad beans	Blueberries	
Vegetarian chili	Blackberries	**SNACKS**
Soybeans	Cherries	Apple Bran Muffins (see recipe on p. 89)

PANTRY	FRIDGE	FREEZER
	Grapes	Homemade Granola Bars (see recipe on p. 90)
BREADS	Grapefruit	**VEGETABLES/FRUIT**
100% stone-ground whole wheat	Lemons	Peas
	Limes	Mixed berries
CEREALS	Oranges	Mixed vegetables
Oatmeal (large flake)	Peaches	Mixed peppers
All-Bran	Pears	
Fibre First	Plums	
Bran Buds	Raspberries	
Red River	Strawberries	

DRINKS	MEAT/POULTRY/ FISH/EGGS
Diet soft drinks	Lean deli style ham/turkey/chicken
Club soda	Chicken breast (skinless)
Decaffeinated coffee	Turkey breast (skinless)
Bottled water	Veal
Tea	Low-cholesterol liquid eggs (Break Free/Omega Pro)

FATS/OILS	
Olive oil	All fish and seafood (no batter or breading)

PANTRY	FRIDGE	FREEZER
Canola oil	**VEGETABLES**	
Margarine (non-hydrogenated, light)	Asparagus	
Mayonnaise (fat free)	Beans (green or wax)	
Salad dressings (fat free)	Bell peppers	
Vegetable oil sprays	Broccoli	
FRUIT (CANNED/BOTTLED)	Cabbage	
Applesauce (no sugar)	Cauliflower	
	Carrots	
FRUIT (CANNED/BOTTLED)	Celery	
Peaches in juice or water	Cucumber	
Pears in juice or water	Eggplant	
Mandarin oranges	Leek	
PASTA	Lettuce	
Fettuccine	Mushrooms	
Spaghetti	Olives	
Vermicelli	Onion	
PASTA SAUCES (vegetable-based only)	Peppers (hot)	
Healthy Choice	Pickles	
Too Good To Be True	Potatoes (small new only)	
RICE	Radishes	
Basmati	Snow peas	

PANTRY	FRIDGE	FREEZER
SEASONINGS	Tomatoes	
Spices/herbs	Zucchini	
Flavoured vinegars/ sauces	Spinach	
SNACKS		
Food bars (Power/ Balance)		
SOUPS **(vegetable- or bean-based only)**		
Healthy Choice		
Too Good To Be True		
Healthy Request		
SWEETENERS		
Equal		
Sweet'N Low		
Sugar Twin		

Appendix II

G.I. Diet Shopping List

PANTRY	FRIDGE/FREEZER
BAKING/COOKING	**DAIRY**
Whole wheat flour	Milk (skim)
Baking powder/soda	Yogurt (fat and sugar free)
Cocoa	Buttermilk
Wheat/oat bran	Cottage cheese (1%)
Sliced almonds	Ice cream (fat and sugar free)
Dried apricots	**FRUIT**
BEANS (CANNED)	Apples
Most varieties	Blueberries
Baked beans (low-fat)	Blackberries
Mixed salad beans	Cherries
Vegetarian chili	Grapes
BREAD	Grapefruit
100% stone-ground	
whole wheat	Lemons
CEREALS	Limes
Oatmeal (large flake)	Oranges
All-Bran	Peaches
Bran Buds	Pears
Fibre First	Plums
Oat Bran	Raspberries
Red River	Strawberries

DRINKS	MEAT/POULTRY/FISH/EGGS
Diet soft drinks	Lean deli style ham/turkey/chicken
Club soda	Extra lean ground beef
Decaffeinated coffee	Chicken breast (skinless)
Tea	Turkey breast (skinless)
FATS/OILS	Veal
Olive oil	Liquid eggs (Break Free/Omega Pro)
Canola oil	All fish and seafood (no breading)
Margarine (non-hydrogenated/light)	**VEGETABLES**
Mayonnaise (fat free)	Asparagus
Salad dressings (fat free)	Beans (green/wax)
Almonds	Bell and hot peppers
Vegetable oil spray	Broccoli
FRUIT (CANNED/BOTTLED)	Cabbage
Applesauce (no sugar)	Carrots
Peaches in juice or water	Cauliflower
Pears in juice or water	Celery
Mandarin oranges	Cucumber
PASTA	Eggplant
Capellini	Leeks
Fettuccine	Lettuce
Macaroni	Mushrooms
Penne	Olives
Spaghetti	Onions
Vermicelli	Pickles
PASTA SAUCES	Potatoes (small new only)
(vegetable-based only)	Snow peas
Healthy Choice	Spinach
Too Good To Be True	Tomatoes
RICE	Zucchini
Basmati	**SOUPS**
SEASONINGS	Healthy Choice
Spices/herbs	Too Good To Be True
Flavoured vinegars/sauces	**SWEETENERS**
SNACKS	Equal, Splenda, Sweet'N Low,
Food bars (Power/Balance)	Sugar Twin (and other artificial sweeteners)

Appendix III

G.I. Diet
Dining Out & Travel Tips

BREAKFAST GREEN LIGHT	BREAKFAST RED LIGHT
Oatmeal	Cold cereals
All-Bran	Muffins
Fruit	Whole regular eggs
Yogurt (fat and sugar free)	Bacon/sausage
Egg Whites—Omelette	Pancakes/waffles
Egg Whites—Scrambled	
LUNCH GREEN LIGHT	**LUNCH RED LIGHT**
Sandwiches —open-faced/ whole wheat	Potatoes (replace with double vegetables)
Meats—deli style ham/ chicken/turkey	Pasta-based meals
Salads—low fat (dressing on the side)	Fast food
Soups—chunky vegetable-bean	Pizza/white bread/bagels
Wraps—½ pita, no mayonnaise	Cheese
Pasta—¼ plate maximum	Butter/mayonnaise
Vegetables	Baked goods

DINNER GREEN LIGHT	DINNER RED LIGHT
Soups—chunky vegetable and bean	Soups—cream based
Vegetables	Caesar salad
Chicken/turkey (no skin)	Beef/lamb/pork
Fish—not breaded or battered	Potatoes (replace with double vegetables)
Salads—low fat (dressing on the side)	Desserts
Pasta—¼ plate	Bread
Rice (basmati, brown, wild, long grain)—¼ plate	Butter/mayonnaise
Fruit	

SNACKS GREEN LIGHT	SNACKS RED LIGHT
Fresh fruit	Chips, all types
Yogurt—fat and sugar free	Cookies
½ food bar (e.g. Balance)	Popcorn, regular
Almonds	Muffins
Hazelnuts	

PORTIONS	
Meat	Palm of hand / Pack of cards
Vegetables	Minimum ½ plate
Rice/pasta	Maximum ¼ plate

Appendix IV

Exercise Calorie Counter

WEIGHT (IN LB):	130	160	200
TIME (IN MIN):	30	30	30
GYM AND HOME ACTIVITIES			
Aerobics: low impact	172	211	264
Aerobics: high impact	218	269	336
Aerobics, Step: low impact	218	269	336
Aerobics, Step: high impact	312	384	480
Aerobics: water	125	154	192
Bicycling, Stationary: moderate	218	269	336
Bicycling, Stationary: vigorous	328	403	504
Circuit Training: general	250	307	384
Rowing, Stationary: moderate	218	269	336
Rowing, Stationary: vigorous	265	326	408
Ski Machine: general	296	365	456
Stair Step Machine: general	187	230	288
Weightlifting: general	94	115	144
Weightlifting: vigorous	187	230	288

TRAINING ACTIVITIES

Basketball: playing a game	250	307	384
Basketball: wheelchair	203	250	312
Bicycling: BMX or mountain	265	326	408
Bicycling: 12–13.9 mph	250	307	384
Bicycling: 14–15.9 mph	312	384	480
Boxing: sparring	281	346	432
Football: competitive	281	346	432
Football: touch, flag, general	250	307	384
Frisbee	94	115	144
Golf: carrying clubs	172	211	264
Golf: using cart	109	134	168
Gymnastics: general	125	154	192
Handball: general	374	461	576
Hiking: cross-country	187	230	288
Horseback Riding: general	125	154	192
Ice Skating: general	218	269	336
Martial Arts: general	312	384	480
Racquetball: competitive	312	384	480
Racquetball: casual, general	218	269	336
Rock Climbing: ascending	343	422	528
Rock Climbing: repelling	250	307	384
Rollerblading	218	269	336
Rope Jumping	312	384	480
Running: 5 mph (12 min/mile)	250	307	384
Running: 5.2 mph (11.5 min/mile)	281	346	432
Running: 6 mph (10 min/mile)	312	384	480
Running: 6.7 mph (9 min/mile)	343	422	528

Running: 7.5 mph (8 min/mile)	390	480	600
Running: 8.6 mph (7 min/mile)	452	557	696
Running: 10 mph (6 min/mile)	515	634	792
Running: pushing wheelchair, marathon wheeling	250	307	384
Running: cross-country	281	346	432
Skiing: cross-country	250	307	384
Skiing: downhill	187	230	288
Snowshoeing	250	307	384
Softball: general play	156	192	240
Swimming: general	187	230	288
Tennis: general	218	269	336
Volleyball: non-competitive, general play	94	115	144
Volleyball: competitive, gymnasium play	125	154	192
Volleyball: beach	250	307	384
Walk: 3.5 mph (17 min/mile)	125	154	192
Walk: 4 mph (15 min/mile)	140	173	216
Walk: 4.5 mph (13 min/mile)	156	192	240
Walk/Jog: jog more than 10 min.	187	230	288
Water Polo	312	384	480
Waterskiing	187	230	288
Whitewater: rafting, kayaking	156	192	240
DAILY LIFE ACTIVITIES			
Children's Games: 4-square, etc.	156	192	240
Chopping & Splitting Wood	187	230	288
Gardening: general	140	173	216
Housecleaning: general	109	134	168
Mowing Lawn: push, hand	172	211	264

Mowing Lawn: push, power	140	173	216
Operate Snow Blower: walking	140	173	216
Raking Lawn	125	154	192
Sex: moderate effort	47	58	72
Shovelling Snow: by hand	187	230	288

Appendix V

Strengthening/Resistance Exercises

Overview

In order to minimize the risk of injury and maximize the impact of exercise, my physiotherapist recommends exercising in the following order:

1. Warm-up

2. Targeted stretching

3. Aerobic/cardiovascular workout activity

4. Strengthening

5. Stretching/cool-down

Warm-up
Warming up is not stretching. Stretching cold muscles can damage them. Warm-ups are procedures to raise your body temperature in preparation for exercise. Methods can vary from a hot shower or sauna to just doing the activity at a slower pace.

Targeted Stretching
I recommend only specific stretching before a workout. For example, if you have a lower back injury, you may need to do exercises that have been prescribed by your health practitioner prior to the workout activity.

Aerobic/Cardio workout
See chapter 8.

Strengthening
I recommend that strengthening be done after the workout activity, when your body is warm and ready for the intensity of the exercise. Strengthening exercises should be done on alternate days to allow muscles to recover. Having two alternating strength programs works well for many people. For example, one day you can do your arm workout and the next day your legs. This also reduces the length of time for each workout. The only strengthening exercises recommended on a daily basis are those for the trunk muscles. It seems that these generally do better if they are worked every day.

The number of strengthening repetitions is determined by your goals. For most of us the goal is to maintain or build muscle mass, to be toned and have the endurance to do everyday activities with less effort. To achieve these goals start at a weight or resistance (Thera-band) level where you can perform fifteen repetitions without feeling overly fatigued on completion. You should repeat this set of exercises two or three times in a session, with a minute rest between each set. You can use the rest time effectively by exercising a different set of muscles and then performing the second or third set later in the workout.

The biggest mistake most people make is increasing their weights or resistance too quickly. This frequently results in an injury and an inability to exercise for several weeks or even months. Many of us make the decision to increase the demands of the program based on the length of time we have been doing the exercise. We assume that because we have been exercising regularly, we must eventually make the program more difficult. This is a false assumption. Though it is true, as we are growing and peaking physically, that we can generally increase the demands on our body, it is not the same once we have peaked. Most people hit their physical peak around age thirty-five. Do not look at your exercise program as one that should get progressively harder, longer or more demanding once established.

How do you know when you are ready to increase the weights or resistance? If you are able to do fifteen repetitions comfortably, I recommend increasing the repetitions to gain what I term a "margin for error." Take the repetitions up in groups of five until you can do thirty. Once you can comfortably do thirty repetitions, then go to the next level of resistance or weight and drop back down to fifteen repetitions. Continue to use this pattern to increase the difficulty of your program as you feel ready.

It is okay to do the same workout for a prolonged period of time. You may want to choose different exercises to prevent boredom, but the program does not have to get harder or more time-consuming for you to continue to benefit.

An excellent book on weight-training is *Strength Training Past 50* by Wayne Westcott and Thomas Baechle. Though it is geared to the fifty-plus age group, it is ideal for anyone.

Strengthening Exercises— Pre- and Post-Activity

Abdominal

1. Lying on your back on the floor, tighten your stomach muscles without moving your back or pelvis. Your back should be held still throughout this exercise. Your stomach will be flat or concave.

2. Feel the contraction with your fingertips, and maintain this position throughout the next stage.

3. Lift one leg to a bent hip and knee position.

4. Bring the second leg up beside it. This must be achieved without your back moving.

5. Slowly straighten one leg horizontally to the floor. Do not allow it to touch the floor.

6. Straighten the knee fully or to the point where you feel you may lose the stomach contraction, then return to the starting position.

7. Repeat fifteen times with each leg, two to three sets.

Hips and Knees

1. Stand on a stair/step or four- to six-inch-high stool.

2. Slowly bend your leg, lowering the opposite foot *almost* to the floor.

3. Progress by increasing the height of the stool.

4. Repeat fifteen times with each leg, two to three sets.

Legs and Buttocks

This exercise is a variation on the traditional "going up on your toes." You should concentrate on slowly lifting your heels off the ground by squeezing your buttocks as well as using your calf muscles. Imagine you are in a vertical shaft and must go straight up the shaft rather than moving forward onto your toes. This uses more as well as larger muscles.

Hold for two to three seconds. Repeat five times, two to three sets.

Thera-Band Strengthening Exercises

Diagonal Trunk Strengthening

1. Stand with your feet shoulder-width apart.

2. Place Thera-Band under your feet. Keep your knees soft.

3. Pull the band from your hip to over the opposite shoulder. Do not let your trunk twist. Keep your elbows straight.

4. Repeat fifteen times on each side, two to three sets.

Biceps

1. Place a single band under one foot.

2. Bend elbow to touch your hand to your shoulder. Keep your wrist straight.

3. Repeat fifteen times with each arm, two to three sets.

Triceps

1. Place your right hand against your chest.

2. Put your left hand against the right.

3. Grasp the Thera-Band in both hands.

4. Pull the left hand straight out from the chest.

5. The closer the two hands are together, the more difficult the exercise.

6. Repeat fifteen times with each arm, two to three sets.

Ws

1. With your hands at your shoulders (90° angle) and Thera-Band behind your neck, pull out to 45-degree angle.

2. Repeat fifteen times, two to three sets.

You may progress with these exercises by doubling the band before going to the next level of resistance.

CAUTION: Elastic resistance should not be continued to maximum fatigue.

Hips and Knees

Resisted Hip Abduction

1. With Thera-Band around leg and opposite end secured in a door jamb, stand sideways from the door and extend leg out to the side.

2. Repeat fifteen times with each leg, two to three sets.

Resisted Hip Extension

1. With Thera-Band around leg and opposite end secured in door jamb, face the door and pull leg straight back.

2. Repeat fifteen times with each leg, two to three sets.

NOTE: To lengthen the life of your Thera-Band, take a piece of nylon webbing (2 feet) and tie it in a loop. Thread and knot the Thera-Band through the loop. Webbing loop and knot are then secured between the door jamb and the door.

Stretching

You should stretch at the end of your exercise program for a couple of reasons. It's calming, helping you to "come down" from the intensity of your workout, and it lengthens your muscles after they've been shortened and tightened while exercising. The ideal time to stretch is when the body is warmed up, either following a workout or perhaps even in the shower. The length of time you should hold stretches varies from ten seconds to one minute, but I recommend holding each stretch for one minute. There is a wide range of books and brochures readily available on stretching exercises; or you could check the Internet.

Some people complain that no matter how much they stretch, they never get more flexible. These people are called "muscle-bound." They're usually strong and even flexible—but in the wrong areas. For example, someone may have an extremely tight hamstring muscle, which is at the back of the thigh. To compensate for the leg tightness, he or she may have increased flexibility in the lower back. People with this type of flexibility often look like a question mark when they try to stretch their hamstring muscles. Without being aware of it, they are stretching their back until it's extremely rounded. Very little of the force they're exerting is going into lengthening the muscle they're trying to stretch. If this sounds like you, ask a health practitioner who understands compensatory muscle patterns to show you how to prevent your body from "cheating." It is very important to learn correct stretching techniques, particularly if you have poor flexibility or if you have a lower back or neck problem. It is also essential to have good trunk strength to prevent any compensatory patterns.

Appendix VI

The Ten Golden G.I. Diet Rules

1. Eat three meals and three snacks every day. Don't skip meals—particularly breakfast.

2. Stick with green-light products only in Phase I.

3. When it comes to food, quantity is as important as quality. Shrink your usual portions, particularly of meat, pasta and rice.

4. Always ensure that each meal contains the appropriate measure of carbohydrates, protein and fat.

5. Eat at least three times more vegetables and fruit than usual.

6. Drink plenty of fluids, preferably water.

7. Exercise for thirty minutes once a day or fifteen minutes twice a day. Get off the bus three stops early.

8. Find a friend to join you for mutual support.

9. Set realistic goals. Try to lose an average of a pound a week and record your progress to reinforce your sense of achievement.

10. Don't view this as a diet. It's the basis of how you will eat for the rest of your life.

GIDiet.com

I'm most interested in your feedback on the G.I. Diet. I would particularly like to hear about your personal experience with the diet and any suggestions you might be willing to share.

You can contact me at **www.gidiet.com**. Every month I will publish some of your responses on the Web site so that everyone can benefit. The Web site will also feature updates on new food choices or relevant medical and exercise developments.

G.I. DIET WEEKLY WEIGHT/WAIST LOG

WEEK	DATE	WEIGHT	WAIST	COMMENTS
1.				
2.				
3.				
4.				
5.				
6.				
7.				
8.				
9.				
10.				
11.				
12.				
13.				
14.				
15.				
16.				
17.				
18.				
19.				
20.				

G.I. DIET EXERCISE LOG

T = Time   D = Distance

DATE	WALKING		JOGGING		BCYCLING		RESISTANCE	STRETCHING	OTHER
	T	D	T	D	T	D	repetitions		

Acknowledgements

While I was writing *The G.I. Diet*, I was also running the Heart and Stroke Foundation of Ontario, which has thirty-six offices and forty-five thousand volunteers and raises over $100 million annually. The book was an enormous drain on my family time, and my wife, Ruth, bore the brunt of my preoccupation. Despite this, she was my cheerleader, culinary advisor and coach. Without her encouragement and support, I doubt if I would have ever completed this book.

Joanne Cullen similarly gave up a considerable amount of her personal time to help me complete numerous drafts. Her contagious good humour and common sense were a great help during some difficult days.

Maureen Dwight, my physiotherapist, who solved my lower back problem with an exercise program that is now a regular part of my life, was invaluable in helping put together the exercise chapters and appendix. Maureen is the director of the Orthopaedic Therapy Clinic in Toronto.

My thanks to my friends at Random House of Canada: Anne Collins for encouraging me to write the book and

Stacey Cameron for keeping me on track with wonderful editing and direction.

Finally, I must thank all my friends and associates who took part in my dietary research. Their feedback provided the focus and essence of the G.I. Diet.

Index

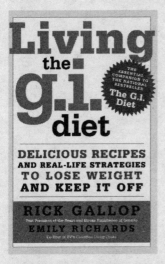